A Little Less Broken

A Little Less Broken

How an Autism Diagnosis
Finally Made Me Whole

Marian Schembari

FLATIRON
BOOKS
NEW YORK

www.flatironbooks.com

All emojis designed by OpenMoji—the open-source emoji and icon project. License: CC BY-SA 4.0

Library of Congress Cataloging-in-Publication Data

Names: Schembari, Marian, author.
Title: A little less broken : how an autism diagnosis finally made me whole / Marian Schembari.
Description: First edition. | New York : Flatiron Books, 2024. | Includes bibliographical references.
Identifiers: LCCN 2024003337 | ISBN 9781250895752 (hardcover) | ISBN 9781250895769 (ebook)
Subjects: LCSH: Schembari, Marian. | Autistic people—United States—Biography. | Autistic women—United States—Biography.
Classification: LCC HV1570.22.S34 A3 2024 | DDC 616.85/8820092 [B]—dc23/eng/20240508
LC record available at https://lccn.loc.gov/2024003337

Our books may be purchased in bulk for promotional, educational, or business use. Please contact your local bookseller or the Macmillan Corporate and Premium Sales Department at 1-800-221-7945, extension 5442, or by email at MacmillanSpecialMarkets@macmillan.com.

First Edition: 2024

10 9 8 7 6 5 4 3 2 1

For Elliot, who sees me as I am.

And June, who's perfect as she is.

Contents

A Little Less Broken

Prologue

I WAS DIAGNOSED ON A FRIDAY. THE HUSHED HYMN OF THE SEA called just outside the window of our vacation rental. On the windy beach below, my husband and daughter chased each other up and down the sand without me, but I'd been waiting months for this appointment, and I couldn't wait a second longer. I needed to know.

With my laptop balanced on the nubby duvet, I settled onto the thin mattress. My teeth chattered, not from the cold of the blustery Oregon coast but from nerves. While I knew it was coming, I also knew the moment Dr. Marsh said the word *autism*, everything would change, the puzzle pieces of my life rearranging themselves into a picture entirely different from the one promised on the box.

There, she'd say. *There you are.*

Why do we so desperately want to label ourselves? All those quirks and habits and idiosyncrasies wrapped in a neat little bow. To be human is so complex, how could we hope to capture it all in a single word? And yet millions of personality tests float around the internet, promising to define us in a dog breed, a Beatles song, or a Disney character reimagined as a piece of cheese. We take them over and over, desperate to see ourselves reflected somewhere other than the isolation of our minds.

I'm a Shiba Inu. "Penny Lane." A triple crème brie Ariel. I've been a thousand people. An adventurous world traveler, an ambitious tech employee, a gregarious roommate. None of them were really me. Underneath the masks lived an overwhelmed, twitchy little girl who—from her very first memory—was told the way she showed up in the world was wrong.

And so she hid.

Once, in middle school, Dad caught me in a lie. I'd probably stolen a twenty from his wallet or gone to a boy's house without a chaperone. He called me into the living room.

"We need to have a chat," he said, patting the couch seat next to him.

I sat in the plush red armchair across from him instead.

The room was crammed floor to ceiling with the kind of art you'd buy at a touristy gallery from a woman with a gray braid wearing quilted overalls. My favorite piece was a three-foot red beaded lizard on the wall next to the fireplace, and I stared at this, unblinking, while Dad interrogated me.

"I can always tell when you're lying," he said, exasperated, when I refused to confess.

"You can?"

"You never look me in the eye." His eyes surveyed me, waiting.

Despite the nausea moving through me, my eyes darted away from the lizard and flicked to his. Making eye contact has always felt like dragging a knife across a dry plate. I shuddered and my skin tensed, as if it had become too tight for my body. I don't remember if he ended up believing me, but from then on, whenever I said anything to Dad I would think, *Look him in the eye, look him in the eye*, as if nothing I said would be believable unless our eyes met. How ironic, that the real lie was the eye contact itself—a habit I trained myself into adopting so I'd appear confident and trustworthy.

And how wonderful it is now, twenty-four years later, in this tiny room next to the beach, to talk to Dr. Marsh after peeling away the layers of myself like old paint.

The most liberating thing about asking a doctor whether you're autistic is you don't have to pretend anymore. After months of research I could surrender to the urges that had been building within me since I was a girl. In most conversations, I miss 75 percent of what the other person is saying because I'm so obsessed with whether I'm making the appropriate amount of eye contact. Not this time. I stared away from Dr. Marsh and toward the closet across from me. The sliding door was open a crack and I itched to close it.

As she talked, I played with the string on my hoodie. It felt almost vulgar to move like this in plain sight without turning my head or covering my face.

I *wanted* her to see me.

That foggy summer morning on the Oregon coast, I finally had a name. I was not lazy or weird or deficient or annoying or disagreeable or moody or sensitive or a liar or broken. After three hours of interviews, fifty pages of surveys, two months of waiting, and thirty-four years of hiding, I finally knew who I was. Who I'd always been.

— 1 —

The Worst Kid in Fourth Grade

MY MEMORY BEGINS IN THE CLASSROOM CLOSET. HUDDLED IN THE corner, I press my back into the coats and lunch boxes, creating a cocoon around my nine-year-old body. To a child, it was more a cathedral than a closet, rectangular and narrow, with high ceilings and bright white walls and a window too high for even a grown-up to reach.

Outside the slatted door were the popular girls, Kim and Carly and Cassie and Katelyn and *three* Katies: Katie K., Katie P., and Katy-with-a-y.

It was Cassie who told me, the other girls giggling behind her. Right before lunch, she approached my desk and said, "We don't want to be your friend anymore."

My stomach dropped to my feet.

"What?" I asked, not confused, but needing a beat to process before I reacted. Some part of me had been waiting for this moment. I had no idea why they'd befriended me in the first place. I was a spunky child, with blunt bangs cut straight across my forehead. There's one picture of me in the summertime, squinting at the camera against the glare of the sun. The girls to my right are clear and blond and smiling, but you can't even make out my face. There I am—pink bike shorts and pink Bugs Bunny T-shirt fading into a dark anonymous blob, my arms tight against my sides as if tensing for a punch. I wasn't particularly pretty or silly or talented, though looking back on it now, neither were they. At least, not the ones who cornered me at my desk that day in fourth grade.

"We don't actually like you." Cassie shrugged. "When we were walking home from school yesterday, Katy-with-a-*y* said she wanted to kick your little Puerto Rican butt." She smirked. I was, at the time, deeply obsessed with Mom's Puerto Rican heritage and talked about it every chance I could. I'd wear Abuelo's guayabera to school and shove tostones in my classmates' faces, but I had a feeling they were talking about more than shirts and snacks.

That's when I ran into the closet, locked the door, and folded myself into the far corner, under a ski jacket with the lift tickets still attached. They followed me and, their voices muffled through the door, listed their grievances.

That was the year I'd read both *Harriet the Spy*, a novel about an inflexible girl with quirky habits and a commitment to espionage, and *A Writer's Notebook*, a thin volume gifted to me by my journalist parents that encouraged young writers to record everything, from our favorite words to snippets of conversation. Author Ralph Fletcher wrote that these notes would "reveal important truths," so I obsessively documented the world around me in the hope that its secrets would become clear.

While folded into the back corner of the closet, I didn't cry or argue or tell the teacher what was happening. Instead, I took out my notebook and transcribed everything they said.

"Can you repeat that?" I shouted from inside the closet. "Talk a little slower?"

"You are a-n-n-o-y-i-n-g," said Cassie.

Tears stung my eyes, but I blinked them back. I focused on transcribing.

You talk too much.
You're no fun.
You're harsh.
You're weird.
We don't like hanging out with you.

My pen shook while I hunched over my notebook, but I recorded every word, as if by studying it later I could pinpoint exactly how to change.

I WOULD HAVE STAYED folded in the closet forever. Maybe part of me still is, like a forgotten glove. Our teacher, Mr. Bacon, eventually realized what was happening and came to fetch me. He led me back to my low tan desk, where my stomach churned like a bag of eels for the rest of the day. When the final bell rang, I walked home alone. A few valiant crocuses poked their heads out of the hard ground.

I lived with my parents and three younger brothers in Old Greenwich, Connecticut, in a house halfway down a quiet, tree-lined street, two blocks from the main thoroughfare. The town itself was wealthy, but in a quaint New England kind of way, the love child of Norman Rockwell and a boat shoe. The houses on our street were modest compared to most of Greenwich; only one had a turret. A smattering of ranch homes squatted between hulking colonials with wraparound porches and tire swings looped over the branches of ancient oaks.

Ours was a tall square box with a hand-painted poster board sign stuck in the lawn that read SLOW DOWN! CHILDREN LIVE HERE! Before the city installed speed bumps, sometimes Mom would stand outside, waving it accusingly at cars that sped by.

As our family grew, my parents built *up*, our home eventually resembling the Weasley house from Harry Potter, leaning to one side from the weight of the expansions and my siblings' relentless noise. Inside, the walls were lime green and royal blue and hot pink, with bright art crowding every wall. In a town known for beige on beige, pearls, and custom marble countertops, our house was where discarded paint cans found their forever home.

Mom was in the living room when I returned from school. At the sight of her, I burst into tears, the front door not even fully closed behind me.

"What's wrong?" she asked.

"My friends—the g-g-g-irls said they never liked me. Th-th-they don't want to be my friend anymore." I collapsed on an armchair and told her everything.

"Ah," she said when I was done. A long, unreadable pause. "What did you do to upset them?"

"I didn't do anything!" I wailed.

All I wanted was to feel the warm weight of her. To have her pull me close, wipe away my tears, and kiss my forehead. To hear her whisper in my ear, "You are wonderful and perfect and those jerks don't deserve you." My need for her comfort was primal, and it broke my heart.

"Honey." She took a pained breath, but her tone was soft and gentle, a genuine attempt to help me. "I think this might be an important lesson for you. I had to learn it when I was your age. You need to be more pleasant with people. You can be . . . harsh . . . sometimes."

Harsh. Cassie had used that word too. I launched my little body out of the chair and shouted, "I just wanted you to be nice to me!"

"You want me to be nice instead of telling you the truth?"

I ran out of the house and into the woods.

OUR BACK LAWN ENDED at a low stone wall, which separated our house from a patch of trees, which separated our neighborhood from a private golf course. My brothers and I would sometimes hike in armed with old egg cartons and fill their dimples with lost balls, which we'd clean with toothbrushes and sell back to wealthy golfers for twenty-five cents each.

Oh, how I fantasized about staying in those woods forever. Not only on this day, but every day.

The woods were always quiet. At home, my three brothers were a tumbling pile of noise. They talked at three times the volume of normal people, usually all at once and with a thunderous crescendo. After school, I could hear them chewing from three floors up, and if I wanted a snack, I'd have to army crawl through the kitchen, dodging Nerf bullets.

Family dinner was a cacophony of yelling, clattering, thumping, and scraping. Despite multiple conversations happening at once, everyone somehow managed to interact with one another. Joe and Sam would argue over which chair was theirs. Dad asked each of us about our day. Antonio got angry because Joe was kicking him. Mom stood up and sat back down twelve separate times before she started eating because she kept forgetting napkins or water or a small, separate dish for the ketchup because *we don't put ketchup bottles on the table.* When Dad eventually asked how *my* day was, I'd look at him, dazed, trying to remember how to answer questions. I'm sure I seemed like any other surly tween with my one-word answer of "Fine," but it was truthfully less about whether I wanted to answer him and more about whether I *could.* And what was there to say anyway? My day was books and trees.

As soon as I'd get home from school, I'd dump my backpack by the front door and rush outside. In the woods, I could be Sam from *My Side of the Mountain,* who ran away to the Catskills to live in a hollowed-out tree. We had a fridge full of food, but that didn't stop me from stealing our chipped enamel salad bowl to collect meadow garlic from the boggy edge of the woodland. I'd come home and boil them in a big pot and serve myself a steaming bowl of "soup." In the woods, I could be Karana from *Island of the Blue Dolphins*. She may have been stranded on a windswept hillside, but she built herself a home out of whale bones and learned to survive on her own, creating a full and quiet life for herself in the wild.

In my woods, at the far edge of the stream was a mess of vining brambles that curved into a dome with an opening the perfect height for a child. Inside was open and airy. When it was dry, I could sit on the mossy earth and imagine myself into someone else entirely.

Even though our block was filled with families, I almost always had the woods to myself. It was my own personal wilderness, and I could pretend I'd never have to return home. I could stay forever, making pancakes out of acorn flour and sleeping under blankets made of leaves. For the characters in my books, loneliness was just another word for adventure.

The trees thickened as I walked in, and eventually my house was out of sight. It was spring and everything was wet and green. My heartbeat slowed, as petrichor entered my lungs and deepened my breath until I was another damp, rustling thing.

I headed to my favorite spot next to the creek, which in my memory was a wide, clear river that cut through the woods. In reality, it's more of a stagnant, muddy puddle. On its bank rested a rock shaped like a whale, with a blowhole on top that filled with water when it rained. I sat there, staring off into the distance like I imagined lonely girls did in books. The afternoon sun poured flickering light onto the water, moving and clear after a spring rain. Willows had started to bud out and dipped their arms into the creek, making divots through the current. I watched for hours. Or ten minutes. Time slowed as if it were already a childhood memory. A splash caught my attention, and I swore I saw the tail end of a small brown creature diving under the water. I was so desperate for these woods to be wild, not merely a strip of trees between suburbia and a golf course.

I wished I could see myself from the outside. *Was* I harsh? Did I constantly correct Kim and Cassie and the Katies? Did I natter on about journal writing and empanadillas, never asking about their interests? I can't tell you with any certainty what kind of kid I was back then. I thought I was curious and imaginative and kind, but I'm not sure that ever came to the surface.

Starved for companionship, I devoured stories about kids who ran away to live in a tree or a museum. If they could do it, couldn't I? When I was in the woods, I didn't feel weird. I was a tree, a rock, a leaf. I was exactly what I was supposed to be.

LATER THAT YEAR, THE assistant principal knocked on our classroom door and whispered to Mr. Bacon, who met my eyes and waved me over.

"Can you please go with Mrs. Ross?"

The class turned their attention to me, and a flush crept its pink fingers up my neck.

I scuttled after Mrs. Ross down the long hallway, which was dim and quiet except for the squeaking of my shoes and the muffled laughter behind the closed door of the Talented and Gifted room. We turned into her office, and she flicked on a humming fluorescent light. I took a seat across from her desk. A sinking feeling gnawed at me, but I couldn't remember what I'd done wrong. If I kept my face neutral, maybe the universe would deliver something innocuous, like a missed permission slip. Or maybe my teachers had realized I was brilliant and should be blowing up rockets with the TAG kids.

For a long, squirmy moment, Mrs. Ross looked at me, eyes narrowed, as if waiting for a confession. I stared at a snag in the carpet.

"Did you call another student a 'rich bitch'?" she finally asked.

"I—"

What to say? That *everyone* called him that? That he lived in an even bigger mansion than everyone else, right on the water? That

I literally knew nothing else about him except that the other kids called him "rich bitch" instead of his name? That one day I said it to his face, as if it *was* his name, not really understanding you're not supposed to do that? I never quite understood why we couldn't say exactly what we thought.

I studied the carpet snag, a gray loop standing at attention.

"Look at me," said Mrs. Ross.

My eyes snapped to hers, but it felt like a dissonant chord. How long did I have to hold this? I counted the seconds as they passed. *One, two, three, four, five*. I flicked my eyes back to the snag.

Before I could answer, she placed both palms on her desk as if she were about to push herself up and said, "Marian, you are the worst kid in fourth grade."

The worst kid in fourth grade.

Worse than Ollie, who deliberately threw kickballs at our heads during recess. Worse than the Katies, who cornered me in a closet.

I wish I could remember what else she said, or *why* she thought I was the worst child out of a hundred, but I left her office sure of one thing: I was broken. Something inside me was inherently flawed and unlovable. The unspoken dynamics of my teachers and my family and my peers would never click into place.

I would have to fake it.

—2—

Third Wheel

I WAS SITTING IN THE TALL CHAIR AT THE KITCHEN ISLAND, DRINKING orange tea with a full tablespoon of sugar, when Dad entered the room and patted the top of my head. I winced at the sound of my hairs scratching against my scalp, so I shifted an inch away from him. He took a sip of my tea and grimaced.

"That's like syrup," he said.

I was too busy reading *Calvin and Hobbes* to answer. My only wish in the whole world was to read a book alone in a quiet house and never once be interrupted.

"I love that you read independently," he said with a smile. Then he just stood there, watching me.

At the sink, Mom washed the endless pile of dishes our family of six refused to load into the dishwasher.

"Do you remember when you were bitten by a horsefly?" Dad asked.

"Nope," I said, not looking up from my comic.

"Well, we were at the playground," he continued, oblivious. "You must have been about three or four. We were still living in Chicago. You know that playground, Chrissy? The one by the hospital?"

"Oh, I don't know, Jim," Mom sighed, her gloved hands submerged in the soapy water.

"Right," he carried on, "so, we'd taken you to the playground and you were in the sandbox and a horsefly must have bitten you, because one second you were playing happily and the next you were screaming, 'Daddy! Daddy! Daddy!' But we left you there to cry." My father grinned and his eyes prodded for mine, but I kept my gaze locked on the book, though I could no longer make out the words. "All the other parents would rush to their kids and kiss their boo-boos, but not us!" His chest inflated like a balloon and practically carried him away.

Dad loves this story. He tells it annually, even now, though the details often change. In another version, I fell and skinned my knee, and I wept on the pavement while I stared horrified at the swipe of blood oozing down my shin. In another, a friend abandoned me in the sandbox, and I cried for her to come back. Dad, a journalist with a popular Family Man column, wrote for the *Bridgeport Post* about this last one: "My daughter, confused and hurt at suddenly losing her friend, called repeatedly after the girl. The friend eventually came back, but for a few moments the pain I felt was worse than any heartbreak."

Regardless of what made me cry, and despite the pain he claimed to feel at witnessing my tears, in each version my parents chose not to comfort me. "To teach you independence," Dad said. "And look at you now!"

AFTER THE CLOSET INCIDENT, it didn't take long for me to find my way into another group of friends, which says less about me being in hot demand and more about the kindness of a girl named Chelsea.

Chelsea had the presence of a freckled giraffe, tall and lanky. Her dirty-blond hair fell down her back in waves, and she dressed as if her parents kept a homestead and practiced some Puritan religion from the 1800s, which was odd because her family was a feral, fantastic group of hippies who smoked in the house and let us call them by their first names.

Near the end of fourth grade, Chelsea approached me on the school playground as I sat alone in another sandbox. "Do you want to be friends?" she asked. And that was that. She folded me into her friendship with an Italian named Giulia, who was short and soft, with a thick accent and even thicker hair that made her look like da Vinci's *La Scapigliata*. Over the following days and weeks, their duo became our trio. On weekends, we had sleepovers and practiced kissing our pillows and choreographed dance routines to Eiffel 65's "Blue (Da Ba Dee)." We rode our bikes around town in the summer. We dressed like Madonna and walked to CVS to buy candy. Once, I cut Chelsea's hair almost all the way off. I meant to give it a trim, but I kept making one side shorter than the other, and by the time I managed to even it out, her previously waist-length mermaid hair was at her chin. (She loved it; her mother did not.) These new friends were the silliest, weirdest people I'd ever met, and with them, I was too.

Then, one day, Giulia told us her family was moving back to Europe. We cried in each other's arms for weeks before Chelsea and I waved her off like war widows.

Like most preteens, we grieved just long enough to replace Giulia with Elena, another European.

Elena walked the halls of Eastern Middle School surrounded by an entourage. Everyone loved her, from the band nerds to the captain of the swim team. She was the rare tween who bridged the gap between the popular kids and the ones who paraded through CVS dressed like Madonna. Elena had shiny hair that always looked like she'd stepped out of a salon.

Regardless of my own unfortunate hairstyle (I had not one but two cowlicks that framed my forehead like parentheses and made me look like an off-brand member of the Backstreet Boys), my social life revolved around Chelsea and Elena. With them, I wasn't alone. They were my lifeline, my connection to other kids—though I never relaxed fully around them either, as if I were playing the part of their friend and never truly connecting with my own needs.

Once, the morning after a sleepover at Chelsea's house, we were tired after staying awake too late watching *Liar Liar*. We'd pushed back the couch to make room for our sleeping bags, which now lay in a tangled pile. The living room windows didn't have curtains, and the early-morning sun streamed into our eyes. Upstairs, Chelsea's brother was doing something that required lots of thumping and crashing, and in the kitchen down the hall, her mom was making breakfast, pots and pans clanging.

Elena, who had the uncanny ability to impersonate Jim Carrey, turned to us and drawled, "Allll righty then!"

I padded into the kitchen to grab a bowl of dry cereal. When I came back, Chelsea was half whining, half giggling.

"Elenaaaaa."

"Allll righty then!" Elena said again with a sly smile.

Chelsea shoved her.

Elena got right up to her face, nuzzling her shoulder before whispering in her ear, "*All righty then.*"

"Oh my god, you're insane!" Chelsea pounced, and they tumbled off the couch and onto the pile of sleeping bags, squirming and shrieking, rolling over each other like puppies.

I stopped behind the couch and watched them. I could see us all from a great height. Oh, there's Chelsea whacking Elena's butt. Oh, there's Elena pulling Chelsea's hair. Oh, there I am off in the corner like a little troll.

I wanted to *want* to join them. To be the kind of carefree person who played easily with her friends. But their laughter made me twitch. The light was too bright, I was tired, it was early, the house thundered with noise. Every sound had been magnified and I could hear every movement: Chelsea's dad scratching his nose in his bedroom upstairs, the run of the shower on the third floor, a toilet flushing down the hall, a car door slamming across the street, an ant crawling along the windowsill.

My brain shouted: *GET OUT.* I wanted to disappear into the floorboards or, better yet, run out the door and back home to my quiet bedroom with my books and my collection of sea glass. If I slipped out, would they even notice?

I couldn't tell you why I didn't want to play. Was I afraid of looking silly? Did I not want to be touched? All I know is that resistance appeared in my body for what seemed like no logical reason. No matter how hard I tried to make myself move the way I thought I was supposed to, I couldn't.

"What are you doing standing there?" Elena called from inside their cuddle pile.

"C'mon, Mare, jump in!" Chelsea said, always the camp counselor.

Gratitude did not wash over me. I didn't want to be noticed. I'd changed my mind; I didn't need a friend in the sandbox. I was perfectly happy alone.

My throat closed and my feet rooted to the spot, as if someone had poured concrete over me. Any lingering energy sucked out of me in a *whoosh*, and all that remained was an angry shell, a voice in my head trying to bully me into participating.

Just jump in, Marian, have fun! This is what girls do. You're such a loser, will you loosen up already? C'mon they're staring at you now; you look like such a weirdo. Jump, Marian, JUMP!

I didn't jump. I stood there on that bright Saturday morning in my best friend's living room, eyes darting for an exit, stuck on the thought that I was not, in fact, like the other girls, and it was only a matter of time before they realized it too.

When their attention on me eventually waned and they turned back toward each other, my body unstuck itself from the floorboards and I moved silently to the couch, where I ate my dry

Kix by the handful and watched in heavy silence as they played without me.

No wonder no one likes you.

I see that girl with her cowlicks and her sleepy eyes trying so hard to be the peppy, energetic, playful kid everyone wanted her to be, and I imagine taking her in my arms like some romance hero and saying, "You are not broken. There is a better, more beautiful word for what you are."

I wish I had known then what I know now: that millions of other girls also experienced the world as if the volume had been turned up to eleven. They too felt like aliens, watching their peers more like scientists than comrades. I wasn't the only child on the planet who didn't want to jump into the thick of things, who pulled away from touch and laughter and light.

Many, many years later I'd learn the word used to describe people like me—quiet and serious and sensitive but no less deserving of empathy and connection.

But I didn't know then, and I wouldn't for another twenty years.

— 3 —

The Rabbit

AT 2:45 WE BURST OUT OF THE GLASS FRONT DOORS OF EASTERN Middle School and squinted into the bright sun. The air was heavy with the smell of hyacinth and cut grass. A lawn mower whirred in the distance. Summer was close.

"Walk home with us?" Chelsea asked.

The walk was nearly two miles, so I usually took the bus, but it was a beautiful day, so I skipped down the front walk with Chelsea and her friends Steph and Jack, which is when I spotted Danny waiting at the end of the path, hands hooked into the straps of his backpack. He smiled when he saw us and lifted a hand. *Oh my god, was he coming too?* My heart flung itself against my chest. I ran a hand through my hair.

Danny had a perfect heart-shaped face, thick eyebrows, and chestnut skin. He wasn't an unruly boy who yelled and ran down the hall, knocking over other kids without a glance back; he wasn't a clown who sat in the back of class making fart noises whenever a girl walked by. No, Danny smelled like Old Spice and played soccer every day after school—he was going to go pro one day. And he always had a serious girlfriend who, on Valentine's Day, would walk to class holding his hand, proudly clutching pink balloons or a stuffed bear with a heart on its stomach. I was, of course, desperately in love.

At thirteen, my default flirting strategy was to completely ignore anyone I thought was cute. I kept my eyes on the ground or engaged in loud, obvious conversation with everyone but him. I could imagine nothing worse than a boy *knowing* I liked him. (Subscribe to my blog for more great dating tips!)

Danny did join us on the walk home, but I stuck close to Chelsea as the five of us walked across the cast-iron bridge on Riverside Avenue, over the train tracks and onto the tree-lined streets that would take us home. Chelsea hopped onto an old stone wall and balanced across the length of it like a gymnast.

"Should we play a game?" she asked, arms straight out on either side of her.

"Absolutely," said Jack.

Our favorite was the Penis Game. Who would be brave enough to shout the word *penis* as loud as possible in the middle of our pristine WASPy neighborhood? Steph, a shy, mousy girl, kicked us off.

"*Penis*," she said, the word barely noticeable under her breath. I giggled.

"Penis," Jack said, at a normal volume.

"Peeeeeenis," sang Chelsea, a little louder, her face flushed.

"PENIIIIIIIIIS!!!!" I screamed at the very top of my lungs. My throat burned. They all burst into laughter and I beamed. They were laughing with me, not at me. I could be the brave one! The loud one! I blinked hard and flared my nostrils.

"Why do you do that?" Danny asked.

I stilled. *Was he talking to me?*

"Do what?" I hitched my backpack higher on my shoulder. "It's just a word, I don't care how loud we say it." If I pretended he was talking about the game, maybe he would drop it. But I knew he wasn't.

"No." He stopped and turned to me.

I let my face go slack and still. *Don't blink don't blink.*

"I mean, why do you do that thing with your face?" He scrunched his nose like Samantha from *Bewitched* and fluttered his eyelids.

"You look like a rabbit," he added.

The group had gone quiet. My brain scrambled and misfired, searching for something funny to say that would break the tension.

At thirteen, I was still under the illusion that most people didn't notice the repetitive movements I made with my face, but I was old enough to subconsciously understand that if they did notice, the polite thing was to ignore it.

Two other girls in our grade had facial tics—Becky and Rachel, who were twins. One afternoon in the crowded, sweaty hall between classes, Becky and I stood outside Ms. Campbell's homeroom, waiting for the bell to ring. Every thirty seconds Becky blinked quick and hard. I looked away, embarrassed for us both, as if I'd walked in on her in the bathroom, pants around her ankles. It was too intimate, and the easiest solution was to act like nothing happened.

There was comfort in that thought, but also fear. On the one hand, I felt protected by the knowledge that people would never call me out. I could blink or flare as often as I wanted, and no one would say anything. On the other hand, I was also starting to realize that my classmates probably did notice and were turning away from *me* in secondhand shame.

But here was Danny asking point-blank: Why? I didn't get to answer because Jack interrupted by shouting, "PEEEEENIIIIIIIIIS!!!" The group broke into relieved laughter, and we continued our trek home.

Why did I do it? It wasn't a choice, really. I blinked and flared because it felt good in my body, like scratching an itch. My eyes needed air, so I'd open them wide enough to feel the cool breeze on my eyeballs, then I'd blink hard, four or five times. Sometimes I'd repeat that sequence a few times, sometimes only once. The nostril flaring was similar. I'd scrunch my nose and flare it. For as long as I can remember, I've had these unusual movements, and for just as long, I've been trying to hide them.

In kindergarten, I sucked my hair. The rough strands in my mouth comforted me, a visceral sensation to focus on, especially when I was bored in class or church or the car to Grandma's. When hair wasn't in my mouth, I walked around with the wet clump slapping against my face.

Mom was constantly trying to get me to quit. "*Please* stop, Marian, that's disgusting," she begged.

Undeterred, I waited until she wasn't looking, grabbed a quick taste, then tucked the wet strands behind my ear.

When I wasn't sucking on my hair, I thought about sucking on my hair. I longed for the scratchy texture on my tongue, the slight tug from my scalp, the gentle, innocuous taste. I have never been still—always fidgeting and picking and blinking and flaring and shifting and rocking—but my body quieted when I had hair in my mouth.

Sometimes now, I watch my daughter rub the top of her lip as she falls asleep, a holdover from when she sucked her thumb, and her slack-jawed expression and the fluttering of her eyelids take me right back to my five-year-old self.

Mom's disgust wasn't enough to stop me, but fear was. In elementary school, I'd been given the book *The Darwin Awards*—a series of stories about stupid ways people die—and one chapter stuck with me.

As the story went, there was a teenage girl who also chewed her hair. One day, she was rushed to the hospital with an extreme stomachache, and the doctors found a bezoar the size of a football in her abdomen. Since hair can't be digested, it builds up, sometimes growing to massive size. The girl didn't survive, and I never sucked my hair again.

Since habits like these don't magically disappear no matter how many bezoar stories you read, my hair sucking was immediately replaced by something my mother hated even more.

I spat. Right there on our kitchen's dark-green linoleum floor. Carpet was better, because then it was absorbed by the fibers and Mom wouldn't bellow across the house, "MARIAN LEE SCHEMBARI NEGRONI, STOP. SPITTING. ON. THE FLOOR."

I'd be puttering around the kitchen, hunting for snacks like eight-year-olds do, and my mouth would fill with saliva as if I'd been presented with a three-tier vanilla cake with rainbow sprinkles and soft swirls of buttercream frosting, then my mind would fill with the thought, *Get it out get it out get it out.*

So I'd let go. My spit would land with a satisfying *splat* and glisten on the floor. Cleaning it never occurred to me—that's what moms were for. It also never crossed my mind to spit into a tissue or the sink. I must have received some satisfaction from seeing it there, part of me immortalized. I was here! I was alive! I would never die! Unless Mom killed me.

Instead, she begged, she cajoled, she bribed, she threatened.

The only solution that worked was growing out of it and on to the next habit.

Around age nine, all my compulsions moved to my face. I started blinking and flaring my nostrils. There's a video of me from the summer of fourth grade during what appears to be some sort of nerd trivia competition. I'm sitting at a long folding table in front of the stage with three other kids. At the podium is Mrs. MacArthur, her face stern, her severe brown bob swinging as she asks us questions, too muffled to hear.

Dad, filming on his old-school video camera, zooms in on my face for the remainder of the five-minute video. My elbows rest on the table and the backs of my hands press into my cheekbones, fingers dangling down my face. I blink three times, sniff, then put both pinky fingers into the sides of my mouth and pull. I blink again, twice, before turning to the girl to my left to whisper something in her ear. When the teacher starts talking again, I fiddle with my necklace. I pull it away from my neck, slide the silver charm back and forth along the chain, then pop the whole thing in my mouth.

In the moments between questions, I am a nervous, twitching thing. When I turn to my teammates it's as if a switch gets flipped. I'm animated and smiley and truly fucking adorable. It's when I'm lost in my own thoughts, not thinking about anyone else around me, that you can see the weird ball of anxiety underneath my baggy blue T-shirt and knee-length jean shorts.

I am still this person.

Depending on what's going on in my life, different comforting movements appear beneath my skin. In high school, at my most stressed and self-conscious, I picked at my face, already a constellation of pimples and scabs. During choir practice, I'd sit in the alto section waiting for my part to begin, ripping at the topography of my skin.

I knew, of course, that you should never touch your face, especially not when you're a hormonal teenage girl, but if I didn't, tweaking anxiety would build in my body and I'd stop being able to focus on Mr. Sawyer waving sheet music at us and all that energy would focus on what my hands *weren't* doing. I felt too still, too exposed. Even though it hurt, the picking soothed me.

In college, I rolled my neck. I'd settle in to study on my creaky futon, but before I could relax into the work, I'd jerk my head back, then roll it side to side until it popped. I'd do it over and over, until my head ached.

In my twenties, I started locking my knees when I walked. I still do this, especially at the beginning of a walk, in the weird limbo between home and the outside world, before I've settled into the rhythm of walking. I head out my front door and down the driveway, turning right onto my suburban street. The trees, the flowers, the houses are all familiar, but it's jarring to leave the safe space of my home, like adventuring into the unknown. For nearly half a block I'll take a step and lock my knee—step, lock, step, lock. I look like I'm jamming out to the Jackson 5 on invisible headphones. Like the other habits, knee-locking is a movement I can control, but it has a calming effect, so I don't.

My family never talked about any of this, maybe because we all did it.

Antonio, the brother right below me, also blinked a lot, and he too has continued this through adulthood. When Sam, the middle brother, was seven, he'd do a little dance as he walked. He'd stop, knock his knees together, snap his fingers, then carry on as if nothing had happened. After doing this a few times he'd end up far behind us. This was a running family joke.

"Hold on, we gotta wait for Sam to finish his dance!"

"Hurry up, Sammy, you're lagging!"

I laughed and teased along with my parents and brothers, but I saw it for what it was. He wanted to stop. He couldn't stop. Something inside him needed to be expressed through the majesty of dance.

Years later, Sam and I talked about it over the phone.

"It was pretty debilitating," he admitted. "It wasn't subtle. It wasn't like catching someone picking their nose. I was literally stopping and spinning in the middle of the street."

"I know, dude," I told him. "I still can't walk without stopping to lock my knees every few steps. I'm terrified everyone can see me. I want to have a nice, relaxing walk like a normal person."

Sam eventually transitioned into facial tics too, plus a few other comforting movements, like rubbing his shirt between his fingers.

Joe, the youngest, is free.

The obvious question here is whether other members of my family are also autistic. While their tics might not, on their own, indicate autism, autism is hereditary, and it wouldn't surprise me if they too find their way to a diagnosis someday.

We received these glorious gifts from Dad. He smells his food before he eats it. Not every bite, and usually not at white-tablecloth dinners—it's more of a mindless thing, while he's eating popcorn and watching a movie.

I lived in New Zealand in my early twenties, and one summer Dad came to visit. I worked for a dairy company that made unbelievable lemon curd yogurt that I hoarded in my fridge and ate straight from the tub. Dad was crashing on my couch, and one night he stayed up late, watching TV and eating through my yogurt stash.

I walked into the living room to say good night, but before I opened my mouth I caught sight of him, small and vulnerable. He dipped his spoon into the tub of yogurt, brought it to his nose for a sniff, then popped it into his mouth.

Watching Dad sniff each spoonful of yogurt, I thought, *That's who I am.* I saw myself in him from a distance, the oddness of our behavior so flagrant against the brown couch cushions. There he was, there I was, alone and awkward, twitching and flaring, stars on the verge of collapse, exploding in a flash brighter than the galaxy.

IN EIGHTH GRADE, I had English with a boy named Adam. One afternoon, the fire alarm wailed through the school. The blaring siren interrupted Ms. Campbell, and the class erupted into cheers. We pushed our metal chairs back from our desks in an unsettling, scraping chorus. Outside the classroom, feet thundered down the hall.

Before I could walk out, I heard a moaning from the back of the room. I turned to see Adam covering his ears, rocking. His aide stood and moved toward him. Adam shoved back his chair and darted toward the window, hands pressing hard into his ears. Then he flew around the classroom, flapping his arms like a trapped bird.

I'd seen Adam hand flapping before, though it wasn't until decades later that I'd understand it. At their very basic level, self-stimulating behaviors, or *stimming*, are repetitive movements we do when we're overwhelmed or excited. Hand flapping isn't the only stim, and autistic people aren't the only ones who do them. Common stims include biting your nails, twirling your hair, jiggling your foot, or cracking your knuckles. Most people have at least one comforting habit, and the most accepted theory is that these physical movements help lower stress, cope with boredom, and relieve excess energy. When neurotypicals do them, we call it *fidgeting*, which is not nearly as pathologized as stimming.

In an autistic person, stimming can involve socially unacceptable behaviors like rocking, bouncing, spinning, repetitive blinking, sniffing, skin picking, and speaking certain words or sounds out loud. Many autistic people say these movements help relieve their stress, as well as simply being enjoyable. The most beautiful explanation I've heard about stimming is by Amelia Baggs in her YouTube video "In My Language," where she describes her rocking, singing, waving, and playing as "being in constant conversation with every aspect of my environment, reacting physically to all parts of my surroundings . . . an ongoing response to what is around me."

Regardless of the reason, these movements can be deeply stigmatizing and isolating when done in public. I've heard from many autistics who were told that their stims were disruptive and to cut it out, but suppressing a stim can cause even more anxiety.

In my twenties, during a therapy session where I begged to be rid of these movements, my therapist asked me, "Have you ever seen a dog get into a fight at the park?"

"Sure."

"And what does he do afterward?"

I thought for a moment. "Well, my dog does this shiver. He's not wet, but it looks like he's shaking water off his body."

"Exactly. He's literally *shaking it off*. It's nature's way of eliminating stress hormones. What if instead of seeing your tics as uncontrollable, you think of them as your body's way of soothing itself?"

I'd never considered these movements as positive.

And I definitely never imagined that Adam and I were experiencing a similar world, expressing our frazzled feelings through physical movement. His overstimulation came out through moaning and flapping and rocking, mine through blinking and flaring and hair sucking and spitting and locking my knees.

When most people think about autism, they think of boys like Adam. Until I was thirty-four, I thought of boys like Adam. I didn't know that autism could look different from person to person. I had no idea what my body was doing or why. Without a word for what was happening, I resorted to internal insults. I was a weird, disgusting rabbit. My tics were a sign hung around my neck in shaky red script that read OUT OF ORDER. They were a visible indicator of something defective inside myself, a physical manifestation of faulty wiring, a clear differentiator between me and humans.

—4—

The Princess and the Pea

WE SPENT SUMMER SUNDAYS AT GRANDMA AND GRANDPA'S HOUSE.
They had a kidney bean–shaped pool with a diving board.

The day would start out fine. Better than fine. Sundays at Grandma's were the height of East Coast summer in the nineties, all green
grass and sprinklers and games of catch on the front lawn under the
shade of a shining red maple, followed by cheeseburgers grilled over
charcoal. Dad's parents lived in the same house where he grew up, a
single-story ranch straight out of the sixties. His sister, Diana, lived
next door, and a stone path connected their two houses through a
gap in the hedge.

Immediately upon our arrival, my brothers and I would tumble
out of the car, tearing off our shirts and shorts and sandals, leaving a
trail of clothes behind us. We didn't stop to greet our grandparents
but bolted for the diving board, which bent and shuddered as we
catapulted ourselves one by one into the air, where for a moment
we flew before flopping into the water with a thundering splash.
We played Marco Polo. Dad and I practiced a synchronized swim
routine. When I was thirteen, I taught the boys how to play a game
called Queen of Sheba, which required that I float lazily in the

blow-up raft across the still pond of the pool while my brothers had to scurry around and obey my every command. "Bring me soda! Fan my face!" Yes, I invented this game, and no, my brothers didn't know that.

Eventually I would abandon them. One day, when Sam was doing flips off the diving board while Antonio cheered and, with no one watching, Joe tried to wriggle out of his orange water wings, I took in a lungful of air before diving deep into the cool blue water. I kicked hard and swam down down down into the deepest part of the pool, down to where the eye of the drain beckoned me and the pressure was a tight embrace. Above, the muffled sound of a splash. The surface tried to pull me back to her, and my fingers scrambled to hook into the drain to keep me there, but the holes were too small and I couldn't get purchase. I had to keep moving, or else I would float to the surface.

In the deep end of Grandma's pool, I was a mermaid and everything was quiet. In the deep, I was alone. It was just me and the rush of blood in my ears, the distant splash of the above world. While the boys practiced their jumps, I swam, coming up for air only when absolutely necessary.

My legs, pressed together into a tail, undulated like a fish. I swam back along the length of the pool to the bright and sparkling shallow end, where the light reflected off the bottom. As my lungs tightened for air, I pushed farther, willing myself to make it. Mermaids didn't need air. The white concrete floor was grainy like sand, and I dragged my fingertips across it, feeling the texture. Down here, the muffled splashes and distorted noises of my brothers were friendly creatures swimming alongside me.

I broke the surface with a gasp and was met with the sudden and amplified voices of my family.

"Why are you swimming like that?" called Dad.

I blushed, face half-submerged in the cool water. "No reason. Just practicing."

He looked at me for a long moment before going back to his book about World War II naval ships.

The boys were still playing and shrieking, but I had become painfully aware of the noise. I might have noticed it earlier, but in the pleasure of summer I'd been distracted enough by my own joy not to notice. But now their shrill voices raked my skin. I hopped out of the pool and dangled my legs in the water, wondering whether anyone would notice if I crawled inside Grandma's cool, dark house for the rest of the afternoon.

Suddenly, I hated everything. I hated the pool, I hated my brothers, I hated my sweet angel grandma, I hated the sun, I hated the summer, I hated my too-tight bathing suit and the wet hair dripping down my shoulders and the thick smell of cheeseburgers and those stupid wind chimes on Grandma's porch.

Aunt Diana hovered over me and asked, "How are those girlfriends of yours? Kelsey and Helena?"

Without thinking I snapped, "You mean CHELSEA and ELENA?!"

I heard myself, I really did, but my actions were no longer mine to control. I watched myself act like a brat, but couldn't everyone hear themselves? They were shrieking! Didn't they feel how their wet hair sent restless rivers down their shoulders?

A swirling miasma of anger overtook me. I couldn't have told you I was overstimulated, or that the world around me had become too much to bear. Nor did I know that an hour in Grandma's quiet house might have revived me enough to dip back into my family.

Instead, I gave one-word answers until Dad snapped at me for being rude. When I laid my towel on the hot asphalt of the driveway to take a nap, Mom shouted across the yard, "You can sleep when you're dead!"

Around six or so, it was time to go home. We piled back into our red Chrysler minivan, but I forgot to call "Bucket seat!" so Sam and Antonio had already claimed the middle row with fearless smirks.

I was too exhausted to antagonize them, so I crawled over their damp bodies and stuffed myself into the wayback next to the vent window. The car was always covered with a fine layer of Cheerio dust, and once Joe had left a cheese stick in the crease of his car seat and, despite Mom's endless scrubbing, the car still smelled rotten and stale. Today, there were extra notes of chlorine and the sweat of boys approaching puberty. I tried not to gag.

Dad backed out of the driveway, paused, honked, and waved at his parents, then pushed in the Movie Tape, a homemade playlist with songs from his favorite Dad Movies™. The first jazzy piano notes from Nat King Cole's "L-O-V-E" filled the car.

The boys' chatter ricocheted off the van's interior like gunfire. I closed my eyes against it and tried to focus on the music, but the lyrics competed with their voices and my brain switched back and forth.

L is for the way

"I'D DROP THE BIGGEST BOMB ON YOU."

you look at me

"NO, MY BOMB WOULD BE SO BIG. IT'D BE BIGGER THAN A HOUSE."

O is for the only

"YOU'RE BOTH WRONG. MY BOMB WOULD BE AS BIG AS A PLANET."

one I see

"MOOOMMMMM! *V* SAM *is* SAYS *very* HIS *very* BOMB *extra* IS AS BIG AS A PLANET!"

I lost it, channeling my very best Big Sheba Energy. "Guys! You are so loud. SHUT. UP."

Sam rolled his eyes in Antonio's direction and laughed. "This is how we talk, get over it."

"Jeez, you're so aggressive," said Antonio.

"Yeah!" piped up little Joe from the seat next to me. He was always relegated to the wayback.

Mom twisted around from the front. "Marian, stop being so sensitive, they're not talking to you."

I swallowed another outburst. *How am I aggressive, but the boys talking about bombs aren't?*

"Fine," I snapped. "Can you at least open the back window? It smells so bad in here."

Without another word, the rear window pushed open an inch, and I pressed my forehead against the glass. I wiggled my nose as close to the crack as I could. It was highway air, full of gasoline and exhaust, but it was better than the ghost of cheese sticks past.

The sky was almost entirely black, the lights from oncoming cars rushing toward me as our van chugged along at exactly fifty-five miles per hour in the middle lane. The cool air snaked through the window, and the rhythm of the lights lulled me into a sort of trance, where I could curl into myself and try to block out the worst of the noise and the smell. But I couldn't block out the thoughts. *Why am I so angry? Why can't I enjoy a beautiful summer day without descending into rage?* I seemed to exist on a different planet from everyone, including my family, and nothing could bridge the gap between who I was and who they wanted me to be.

Mom sometimes jokes that she has two different families. "I'm the mother of three boys, but on other days I'm the mother of an only daughter."

It doesn't hurt my feelings when she says this, because it feels true, and nowhere was that more apparent than when my brothers were having fun together while I was tucked into some corner grimacing. There were my brothers—fun affable guys with big personalities and bigger voices—and there was me, quietly off in my own fantasy world, annoyed by anyone and anything that took me out of it.

When I was eight, Dad wrote an essay for the *New York Times* about how raising the boys fulfilled his childhood dream of having a brother. "They go to bed, one in the top bunk, the other in the bottom," he wrote. "By morning, they are in one bed, curled up

around each other like puppies in a box." The essay ends, "I sometimes think that the greatest thing I have ever done is to help create
these brothers. We had another child last year, and for the third time
in a row, it was a boy. The bottom of his crib is already cracked from
the weight of his older brothers, who climb in to play with him. I
am surrounded by brothers. It is better than I ever imagined."

Dad loved having a daughter, but I was separate, a treasure in a
box, alone, to be admired, while Antonio, Sam, and Joe were a ragtag
bunch of best buds. Technically, they are three distinct people, but
they are also a unit. "The Boys," we called them, and the designation
stuck, even now as they enter their thirties.

Antonio is the oldest, born three years after me. The day after his
birth, I stationed myself at his bassinet, singing "Rock-a-Bye Baby"
and patting his wrinkly old-man face, which squinted at me in the
fluorescent hospital lights. When he scrunched up in unhappiness,
I turned to my parents and said in my high-pitched girl voice, "The
baby is crying. Daddy, the baby!" In my mind, their parental instincts were no match for my sisterly ones.

Antonio grew into the kind of baby pictured on the diaper
package—a perfect cherub with a squishy round face and soft curls.
My job was to push him around on his plastic ride-on train. On
Christmas, when he opened his gifts from our parents, I shouted,
"Merry Christmas, Antonio!" as if three-year-old me had gone to
the store with a wallet and purse to request their finest Corn Popper
push toy.

Our middle brother, Sam, was born eighteen months later, and
my family refers to them as Irish twins. They shared a room, but while
Sam was young, I crawled into his bed at night to read him stories.

When Mom got pregnant once again, I prayed for a sister. On
Thanksgiving of that year, the day she went into labor, my aunts and
uncles hunted through the turkey carcass for the wishbone before
presenting it to me like a crown on a cushion, knowing exactly what
I wanted. I would take every precaution I could.

When Joe entered the world, Dad shouted from behind his hulking video camera, "It's a boy!"

"A boy? You have to be kidding me," Mom said, with a spent laugh.

"Marian must have uncrossed her fingers," said her sister Lee, who had stood by her side coaching her through Natural Childbirth Number Four.

In the beginning, it didn't matter that Joe was not a Josephine. He had a swirl of hair on top of his head like a cartoon baby, and for the entirety of his first year I changed his diapers, fed him, and bounded up the stairs every fifteen minutes to watch him nap in his swing while Mom and Dad ate dinner. I brought him to show-and-tell and begged my parents to let him sleep in my bed. When they said yes, I tucked his baby body into mine and sang him to sleep, my repertoire consisting entirely of *The Little Mermaid* soundtrack. In most of our family photos during this time, Joseph is bundled in my arms, my eyes focused on him instead of the camera.

By the time he was one, Joseph belonged to my brothers.

When I was young, it was easy to pin my differences on being the only girl in a family of boys. *Of course Marian would rather read than play basketball with her smelly brothers. Of course she's snipping at them from the back of the car, she's the bossy big sister.* My gender was the easy-to-explain outward sign of the internal otherness we all sensed, and so that otherness was easy to dismiss. Most of the time.

Occasionally, it drifted to the surface. Dad wrote about it in his essay, Mom expressed it when she talked about us as separate families, and I felt it in the back seat of our minivan and seated at the family dinner table and in the quiet of Mom's bedroom as she brushed my hair.

IN FOURTH OR FIFTH grade, my cousin Lorea and I were sitting on the carpet of Mom's bedroom, our backs stamped to the edge of the couch, while our respective mothers brushed our hair. Lorea's was straight and glossy, and she sat still while Titi Cathy brushed it to a shine. My hair is, and has always been, thin and curly. It snags if you look at it wrong. Johnson's No More Tangles was gripped between Mom's knees as she yanked the brush through my knots. I cried. I pleaded. I leaned away from the brush at a gravity-defying ninety-degree angle.

Exasperated, Mom let her hands fall to the couch, and she watched her older sister glide the comb (a *comb*!) through Lorea's hair. Lorea's legs were crossed and her hands rested gently on her knees like a Gaia statue. Mom pointed at her with the brush, as if I hadn't noticed the difference.

"See?" she said. "Lorea isn't whining. It's not hurting her. You're making this harder on everyone. Why can't you be more like your cousin?"

I didn't know why. Each jerk of the brush felt like a hundred needles were being hammered into my hairline before being dragged down the length of my scalp. Despite my best efforts, each tug seemed to be tied to the tear ducts in my eyes. Tug, tear, tug, tear, until my eyes were red and my face was a snotty mess. Did I feel sensations that Lorea didn't, or was I badly behaved? My hunch was the latter. I clenched my jaw and tried to be like my cousin.

The answer to what happened in Mom's bedroom—and in the back seat of our crowded minivan and a thousand other micro-movements during which I was consumed with physical discomfort over sensations no one else seemed to notice—is so much simpler than I imagined. Simpler because I had internalized the names I was called—sensitive, moody, irritable, difficult—but they never felt accurate to my experience. What I felt was pain. Which of course makes sense now, given that I was experiencing a classic sign of autism: sensory overload. The *DSM-5* (the current, fifth edition of the *Diagnostic and Statistical Manual of Mental Disorders*) describes this as "hyperreactivity to sensory input," and it can include negative reactions to specific sounds or textures.

The experience of sensory overload is wildly varied, as are its triggers. For me, it's usually high-pitched sounds or multiple sounds happening at once, like going to a pep rally in a crowded gym or my brothers talking while music is playing. But it can also be the texture of a dry Oreo cookie, a nail file, underwire bras, wool and tags and seams on my skin, and, of course, anything involving my hair.

Hair care presents a sensory minefield. Not only does brushing it feel like an army of fire ants crawling across your scalp, but so does having it swing by your ears, touch your shoulders, or shed a single strand onto your bare arm somewhere you can't see or easily grab. Blow-dryers are too hot and too loud. Hair product is too sticky. If you decide not to style it and put your hair up, you'll get a headache. And if you drive, the feeling of a bun or ponytail touching the car's headrest can be so distracting that driving becomes dangerous. I've spoken with dozens of autistic women who almost universally shared war stories about having their hair brushed. "As a child I would scream bloody murder whenever my mom brushed my hair," one woman told me. "Even now, if someone accidentally tugs on my hair, I get so irrationally angry that I will cry or lash out." As adults, many autistic women wear their hair short to avoid the nightmare altogether, but that requires a trip to the salon where you must fight the urge to run away after a trickle of water gets in your ear or a wisp of freshly cut hair sneaks under the collar of your cape.

And that's just hair.

Don't get me started on clothes—itchy fabrics, too-loose fabrics, too-tight fabrics, buttons on jeans, underwire, underwear, tags, seams in socks, socks period. There's a reason entire companies exist to serve the clothing needs of autistic people, though the vast majority of these are for children, as if autistic children don't grow into autistic adults.

Then there's sound. Light. Taste. Smell. Each sense an open window during a hurricane.

Ira Kraemer, a writer, consultant, and advocate known online as the Autistic Science Person, calls this sensory *pain* as opposed to sensory *overwhelm*. "Loud noises feel like my eardrum is being stabbed with a knife," they wrote in a 2021 blog post. "It's the same physical pain neurotypical people would experience if someone blew an airhorn right next to their eardrum. For me, I get this same pain from vacuums, dishes clinking, restaurant kitchens, lawn mowers, buses stopping, and more." Ira's choice of the word *pain* is deliberate, to erase the implication that we're making it up or exaggerating. Because the problem, of course, is that using the word *sensitivity* can bring a knee-jerk response from others who think we must be overreacting—especially when we are girls and other marginalized folks who were raised to believe that the only way to survive is to shut up and play nice.

Like me, Ira was called annoying, difficult, and "too much." Other autistics I interviewed confessed that when they complained about tight socks or itchy tags or too-bright lights or the humming of a lawn mower five houses down, they were told, "Don't be so dramatic."

> *The world doesn't revolve around you.*
> *You're such a drama queen.*
> *You're like the princess and the pea.*
> *You can't possibly hear that, smell that, taste that, feel that.*

But unlike the princess and the pea, our sensitivities are seen not as a sign of sophistication, but as a burden to the people around us. We're ignored, punished, or teased when we speak up, so we eventually learn to endure our pain, turning the abuse on ourselves. *I must be weak*, we think. *I must be broken.* This internal language and "pushing through" can lead to injury or illness. In one Twitter thread, an autistic woman said she grew up hearing that she was weak, "Which of course led to me walking on ten broken toes for five years, thinking 'walking is painful because I'm just weak.'"

Another woman wrote, "As a child I spent a lot of time crying out in stomach pain. My family ignored me. Said I was doing it for attention and that I was spoiled and lying. I learned to hide it. Turns out I had celiac and I didn't find out until I was thirty-two."

While no one really knows why autistic people are so sensitive, there's a hypothesis about why those sensitivities can be triggered so easily. The Intense World Theory of autism, developed by researchers Kamila and Henry Markram, suggests that autism isn't just a differently wired brain but a brain with *more* wiring. In other words, supercharged. The Markrams argue that all of autism's more socially unacceptable symptoms, such as meltdowns, difficulty socializing, and a perceived lack of empathy, are simply due to the pressures and distractions of living in a constantly overwhelming world. Science journalist Maia Szalavitz wrote about this theory for the blog *Matter*: "Imagine being born into a world of bewildering, inescapable sensory overload. . . . Your mother's eyes: a strobe light. Your father's voice: a growling jackhammer. That cute little onesie everyone thinks is so soft? Sandpaper with diamond grit. And what about all that cooing and affection? A barrage of chaotic, indecipherable input, a cacophony of raw, unfilterable data."

And that data is only increasing its pressure on us as our world becomes more crowded and frenetic. In her stunning memoir *The Electricity of Every Living Thing*, Katherine May wrote that she might not have been so strange in a previous era, in "a quieter world . . . without the whine of mobile phones and the ceaseless electronic drone of voices from the radio and the TV; without the noisy surges of hand driers and the bleeping of train doors; without the flat plastic unknowable surfaces and the dry-air containment of office life; without pulsing lights and the ceaseless sense of personal availability."

This unrelenting sensory environment is debilitating because autistic people have more difficulty adjusting to a stimulus over time. My neurotypical husband can sit in his office and focus on work even though cars speed down our street and there's light construction happening next door and a dog is barking five houses down. After a few minutes, it all becomes background noise, his brain doing its job to admit only the most important stimuli, like when I yell at him from downstairs to ask if the car keys are in his pocket again. On the flip side, the autistic brain operates as if everything is important. After an hour at my own desk, I still flinch when a car sloshes down the wet pavement outside my window or when our neighbor Wilson starts hammering at his roof again. I hear my husband upstairs typing and every shift he makes in his desk chair. Regardless of how much time passes, my brain assumes it's *all* crucial.

Here's the good news. At thirty-six, I now understand what's happening and why. I can pull out my noise-canceling headphones and turn on my white noise playlist, which drowns out everything but the voice in my head, allowing me to do what I do best—hyperfocus on my interests for hours at a time.

The bad news is that you can make accommodations only if you've identified the problem. Neither I nor my parents had the language to talk about what was happening, so at thirteen, all I knew was what I was told, and there are only so many times you can tell a girl she's broken before she starts to believe it.

—5—

Eggshells

TO HONOR THE OCCASION OF MY PRESBYTERIAN CONFIRMATION,
Mom gifted me with a small stone cross coiled with vines and pink
flowers, which she hung above my bedroom door. It was up there
only a month before we had to superglue it back together.

The night it happened I was doing my math homework at the
kitchen table, working on a math assignment. Mom, trying her best
to help, sat across from me, waiting.

"I don't understand this!" I wailed.

"Here, let me take a look." She swiveled the paper toward her.
"Okay. It's been a while since I've done algebra, but do you see how
the x does the supination to the y?"

I didn't. The shapes on the page looked like squiggles made
by my five-year-old brother. I tried to catch the numbers with my
mind, but my brain wouldn't cooperate, and the problems kept flit-
ting away and vanishing into the air.

"Marian, pay attention," she snapped.

"I am!" Tears stung my eyes and I rubbed them away. How embarrassing. Crying over *math*. I bit the inside of my cheek to stop
myself from a hiccuping sob.

Mom pointed to a line running up across the page. "Here," she tapped the paper. "This intersects with the praxis, and all you need to do is dinglehopper the arbitrator and there you go! Can you tell me the answer now?"

"Um . . ." *The dinglehopper and the arbitrator the dinglehopper and the arbitrator . . .* Nope. Nothing. Completely and totally blank.

Mom was staring at me.

I squeezed my eyes shut.

"It's five," she said with a defeated sigh.

"Five," I repeated.

She slid the paper back toward me and I wrote *5* in careful pencil. I glanced at the next question.

$I(n)=(n4)+-5n3+45n2-70n+2424 \cdot \delta 2(n)$
$-3n2 \cdot \delta 4(n)+-45n2+262n6 \cdot \delta 6(n)+42 \delta 12(n)$
$+60n \cdot \delta 18(n+35n \cdot \delta 24(n)-38n \cdot \delta 30(n)$
$-82n \cdot \delta 42(n)-330n \cdot \delta 60(n)-144n \cdot \delta 84(n)$
$-96n \cdot \delta 90(n)-144n \cdot \delta 120(n)-$ 🍶 ⧗n✦⊞ ▯ 🗁 ☎

Inside my brain, a wall slammed shut. I scanned the worksheet and saw thirty more questions, each harder than the last.

Oh god, and there was a *back*.

My head fell like a cannonball to the warm wooden tabletop.

"Up and at 'em, Marian! I have other things to do."

Outside the kitchen window, beyond the green-and-white striped valances, it was getting dark. Mom looked tired, her normally bright eyes dull and droopy. She was in her bathrobe, and the kitchen was a mess, and since no one ever cleaned it but her, she had a long night ahead. I, however, only cared about going to my room and crawling into bed to read my new book about a headstrong princess who ran away from her castle to live with dragons.

The moment I thought about my cozy bed and remembered I had thirty problems swimming before me, another wall slammed shut, cutting off my ability to form words, to explain exactly where I was confused. Mom's eyebrows knit together, and I felt an added squeeze of pressure. *Focus*, I told myself. It didn't help. No part of me understood the shapes on the page.

"Marian—" Mom prodded.

"STOP IT!!!!" I shoved myself back from the table, grabbed the wooden chair between us and hurled it toward her. "JUST STOP IT!" Mom dodged backward and the chair clattered sideways to the floor. The words ripped up my throat. "I DON'T UNDERSTAND. I DON'T UNDERSTAND ANY OF THIS."

Without pausing to turn back, I sprinted through the dining room and up the stairs.

When I made it to my bedroom, the exertion only agitated me further, anger careening through me like shrapnel. I wrenched open the door, flung my body around it, and slammed it closed with every ounce of my thirteen-year-old strength.

The sound echoed through the quiet house. My cross flew off its hook and crashed to the floor, breaking neatly in two.

THIS KIND OF THING happened all the time. My childhood bedroom was a memorial to things I'd thrown or smashed or flung off their shelves in fits of what I always thought was rage. A square desk clock with a crack down one side, thanks to the night I'd heaved it across the room. A framed photograph of Mom and me sitting on a log, its glass missing after I'd swiped it off the shelf in one long sweep.

A hole in the drywall next to my rumpled pink bed.

Mere weeks after my parents had installed a phone in my room, I was sitting on my bed talking to my boyfriend Danny (yes, the

Danny who questioned my nose scrunching—he was, unsurprisingly, a terrible boyfriend), cord trailing across my bed. Most nights we argued. He would twist my words into new meanings and spit them back at me. After a particularly heated conversation, I was midargument when I heard the abrupt interruption of the dial tone. He'd hung up on me. All my pent-up words roared through me and I bashed the phone receiver into the wall—once, twice, three times—until it made a perfect round hole the size of a fist.

My feelings didn't have enough space inside my body. All my attention would narrow into a pinpoint of rage, then balloon so big it needed to escape through my throat and hands. Mostly I took my anger out on things, but sometimes, on very unlucky days, there was a person in my way.

Back in fourth grade, right before summer break, I was standing near the long, low bookshelves in our classroom when I slapped Cassie hard across the face. I have no memory of what we were talking about or why I hit her, but that same squeezing tension is still vivid inside me—all that frustration and confusion with nowhere to go. I hit Dad once too. Sometimes my brothers. Danny twice. Of course, as a white person I could get away with hitting another student with zero consequences, and I'm certain I wouldn't have had that same luck had my skin been darker.

Throwing the chair or slamming the door or smashing a hole in the wall relieved the steam like opening the lid of a pressure cooker. It felt good to destroy, even though I'd later look around at other kids and wonder why none of them seemed to be so easily triggered by things like friendship conflicts or homework struggles.

What is wrong with you? No one else acts like this. Get it together.

But you can't bully yourself into a new personality. Without understanding what was happening to me, I felt the rage overtake me again and again. Mom's go-to phrase was, "I feel like I'm always walking on eggshells around you."

My response, though I never said it out loud, was, *How do you think it feels to be the egg?*

FOR YEARS I THOUGHT I had an anger management problem. In my twenties, therapists used the phrase *emotional dysregulation*, but that language never felt quite right either. Sure, there were times when I was *dysregulated*, but those feelings were precursors to the instant when I exploded into violence, rather than the entire experience.

What was really happening, I know now, was an *autistic meltdown*. Meltdowns happen when our mental capacity exceeds its limit and we temporarily lose control of our behavior. Autistic meltdowns usually happen after continued, inescapable exposure to sensory triggers or cognitive challenges. A meltdown is an intense and involuntary response to an overloaded nervous system. Colloquially, the word *meltdown* also describes the cataclysmic overload of a nuclear reactor, which is my favorite way to explain the devastation of the experience. When I'm having a meltdown, my skin gets tight and my mind goes blank. My body reacts without my consent. I slam my hands on the table or scream so loud my throat hurts. Like a nuclear meltdown, the temperature inside me increases until all systems fail, and the only thing to do is run for cover.

I'm not the only late-diagnosed autistic person to mislabel a meltdown as rage, bad behavior, or poor impulse control. One woman told me, "I thought I was having panic attacks or fits of anger where I would throw stuff. I experienced this all the time as a child and was accused of being on drugs."

Meltdowns can look different from one autistic person to another. For me, they looked like fury and violence—throwing, slamming, breaking, hitting. Sometimes, I would cry so long and so hard that the capillaries below my eyes would hemorrhage, causing a smattering of small red freckles that would last for days. Some autistic people will self-harm, thrash, and flail their limbs, while others will swing hard in the other direction and disengage completely into a shutdown.

A few months after my diagnosis, I was scrolling through an online support group for other late-diagnosed autistics and found endless stories from women who'd always wondered why they exploded after the smallest blips. One story was from Amy, who was sitting in front of her computer one day while on the phone with her doctor's office, struggling to set up an appointment, when she received a cancellation email for a flight she'd been looking forward to. "I just broke down," she wrote. "I started shaking, sobbing, then pounding on the carpet with my hands and letting out broken screams."

I remembered an evening nearly ten years prior when my landlord had sent an email requesting an additional monthly rental fee for the items she was keeping in our apartment, including a bookshelf that was too big to move, glued-on mirrors, and the bathroom towel bars. It didn't make any sense; how could you charge extra for permanent fixtures? My husband, who is neurotypical, was irritated by her request but carried on reading his book after I showed him the email. I, however, felt that pressure appear in my chest. My thoughts spiraled as I mentally adjusted our budget, while trying to figure out the best way to communicate with her without coming across as harsh. What I wanted to say was: *Either take your personal items out of our apartment or let us keep them. I don't want to rent your towel rack, Sabine.* Instead, I ran into our living room and screamed, loud enough for the entire building to assume I was being murdered. I collapsed onto all fours and howled, hot tears streaking down my face. I arched my back in a desperate attempt to push the grief and confusion out of my body. A magazine lay on the floor and I grabbed it, smacking it limply against the back of the couch.

Amy wrote that when she feels powerless, she has to vocalize her rage and frustration. "I must sound insane," she added.

When I read her post, it was the first time I realized I *wasn't* insane. I imagined Amy in her room, pounding the carpet over a canceled flight. I imagined sitting next to her in quiet company, gently letting her know she wasn't alone. I imagined her next to me in Sabine's dingy, overpriced apartment, witnessing the woman I was and not looking away.

In her book *From Anxiety to Meltdown*, autistic author Deborah Lipsky outlines two types of meltdowns: cognitive and sensory. They're identical on the outside, but their triggers are different. A cognitive meltdown can happen when we're given unclear instructions, when we're frustrated by miscommunication, or when an event goes off script—like a flight cancellation or an unusual request from a landlord. Lipsky compares this to a computer crash:

> *Have you ever when sending an email hit the send key and watched nothing happen? If you are like me (very impatient) or a new computer user you hit the key again. Still nothing happens, so in frustration you hit the send key twenty times in rapid succession. The little arrow icon becomes an hourglass and on the top of the screen pops a message that your computer is not responding. In effect the computer froze because you didn't give it time to process the initial request, it then didn't understand what you were asking, so you "badgered" it to move forward by continually pressing the send key. The only way to get it responding again is to shut off the computer and restart it so it can reboot. This is very similar to what happens in the autistic brain during a cognitive meltdown. The brain becomes so cognitively overloaded it can't function anymore so it "shuts down" and the instinctual self preservation mode takes over. We have no control at that point.*

Meltdowns can also be triggered by sensory factors. Most autistic people regularly experience some form of sensory overload, but when we're in an environment that continuously bombards our senses without relief or means of escape, our bodies eventually stop being able to tolerate it and we move into meltdown mode.

A meltdown is the response to an unmet support need. The problem is, undiagnosed autistic women rarely get those support needs met because the world clobbers us with the message that if we speak up, we're selfish, naggy, hysterical, bossy, weak, childish, or shrill. "Stop being so difficult!" is the soundtrack to our childhoods, the refrain worming its way into our psyches until we silence ourselves before anyone else can, pushing through the unpleasantness until we snap.

Social psychologist Devon Price, who is autistic and transgender, wrote in *Unmasking Autism* about the summer he went to sleepaway camp and was disgusted by the texture of the food. "[I] went into a full-blown, sobbing meltdown over it. I got reprimanded for being a picky eater and a crybaby, and was forced to sit at the table all evening, until I gulped some cold ravioli down."

Imagine what might have happened had Devon been given an alternate safe food or, at the very least, the option to skip dinner that night. What if, instead of being scolded for pickiness, he'd been validated and spoken to with kindness and empathy? "That ravioli is freaking you out, huh? Are there any safe foods you can stomach right now, or would you like to skip dinner tonight? Tomorrow we're having pizza."

Same effort, *very* different results.

Like most parents and caregivers of undiagnosed autistics, my parents were at a loss as to how to handle my anger, and I don't think they had the emotional tools to handle their own either. I wouldn't say my family is repressed, but there wasn't an eager curiosity about our feelings either. You behaved or you didn't; there was no in-between. The idea of an "unmet support need" would have sounded like whiny navel-gazing. After an incident, my parents' go-to tactic would be a punishment, lecture, or both, after which we'd move forward and act like it would never happen again. Their best attempt at diverting a meltdown was to tease me, hoping that would lighten my mood. When Mom sensed an attitude swirling in me, she'd give Dad a knowing glance and a wink before stage-whispering, "Marian's in one of her moods."

The dismissal only served to pull me more tightly into myself. I was unreasonable. My anger was wrong. No one else ever experienced this but me. And since there was never a safe place or time to let go, the release would come when I least expected it, a sudden storm that pummeled us all.

I would eventually learn to control the rage, but not by denying the feelings or pretending they weren't there. The secret that stopped the screaming and the throwing and the hitting was understanding *why*.

The rage didn't end until the mystery did.

—6—

Main Character

I WAS SIXTEEN WHEN I READ THE BOOK THAT WOULD CHANGE THE direction of my life.

The beige cover was straight out of 1998, like a dELiA*s catalog for bookish girls, featuring an illustrated collage of travel mementos: a passport, a luggage tag, a dried yellow daisy, a photograph of a pretty brunette in a puffy red vest and brown boots, lounging on a green hillside framed by rugged peaks. It was called *Bloomability* and written by Sharon Creech, whose many worn novels weighed down my bookshelf until the cheap laminate bowed in the middle.

The story follows Dinnie, an American girl who's arrived at a boarding school in Lugano, Switzerland. Dinnie refers to Switzerland as her "second life." After years of bouncing from one place to another, always the new kid and the oddball, she easily integrates into a group of expats, who are all foreign and curious in this new place. These kids think it's cool to study and try out for the school play and go to Florence to learn about art history. "In some of my other schools," she says, "it had been cool to go to the mall or to the movies or parties. It was cool to take a test without studying. It was cool to drink and smoke and swear. Those things were definitely not cool at this school in Switzerland."

By the end of her year abroad, Dinnie has blossomed. She ate dripping gelato in cobblestoned squares and romantic avenues flanked by cypress trees, to the soundtrack of the bells of St. Abbondio. She watched men lead cows across the green hills. She learned to ski—because of course her international school hosts a two-week ski term in St. Moritz, where academics take a back seat to lessons on the snow. Dinnie is finally home.

I devoured *Bloomability* under the covers of my twin bed, tucked underneath the eaves of my attic bedroom like the characters in so many other YA novels right before being called to some greater purpose. It wasn't so much Dinnie herself who drew me in but the empty vessel of her life, into which I could pour my own fantasies for the future.

It was my junior year of high school, and every morning I boarded the 6:55 a.m. bus outside my neighbor's house. The only available seats were in the middle of the bus, wedged between the raucous rows of popular kids at the back and the furtive freshmen in the front. Most mornings, I eavesdropped, pressing my ear against the cracked brown vinyl seat in front of me and transcribing into my journal whatever Heather or Jamie or Sabrina said, exactly as I'd been doing since fourth grade.

Despite pinning my hopes on a fresh start in high school, my ability to fit in was no better than elementary or middle school. Both Elena and Giulia had moved back to Europe, and Chelsea had moved on to the popular crowd, exchanging her hand-me-downs and mermaid waves for crop tops and flat-ironed hair. When it was the two of us, we occasionally connected like we used to, but at school she was trying on a new side of herself, and I didn't recognize the distant way she talked or the vacant smile she wore as she took long strides down the hall, my small racing steps barely able to keep up. For the first few months of freshman year, I didn't take the hint and hovered around her new friends like a neurotic hummingbird. I never knew quite what to say, so I'd either hang back in stony silence or force my way into the conversation by blurting something wildly inappropriate, argumentative, or both.

I studied the people around me and tried to mimic their personalities, but I couldn't quite nail the tone of voice or giggle that made someone like Chelsea blossom, while I remained the same prickly weed.

My frustration turned to irritability, and I eventually stalked down the halls alone. More than once, kids mistook me for a teacher.

This was the same year I wandered downstairs one evening at home, and before I rounded the corner into the kitchen, I heard Mom talking to Adriana, our family's bubbly, always-dancing twenty-year-old au pair whose laugh sounded like a pot of boiling water.

"If I had another daughter," Mom was saying, "I would want her to be like you."

That week I bought a brand-new journal from CVS with a pale-green cover framed by cherry blossoms. On the first fresh white page I wrote—

Gratitude Journal

I want to start this because I don't want to end up lonely, mean, and depressed. I want to be a pleasure to be around.

Goals:
1) Be more positive!
2) Smile.
3) Create a wider circle of friends.

Ten years from now I want to be able to look back on my high school years and not see hate.

Later entries revert right back to negative self-talk, calling myself a bitch on approximately seventeen different occasions.

I wasn't like the other sixteen-year-olds. I still escaped into the woods after school to crunch through dried leaves in my New Balance sneakers and sit on my whale rock. I daydreamed about the smell of libraries and moss and old stone churches. I spent weekends wandering the neighborhood with my notebook and wrote down the addresses and descriptions of the most beautiful homes I passed, the ones with purple morning glory wrapped around their mailboxes or old stone walls drenched with ivy. I'd hurry back to my room, breathless and windswept, the smell of boxwood hedges and lilac still lingering, to write stories about the happy families I imagined inside.

When I read *Bloomability*, the first thought that crossed my mind was: *A Swiss boarding school . . . That's the answer! This will fix everything!* I wasn't friendless or angry; I was just in the wrong place. I should be wandering the streets of some cozy medieval city, practicing a new language, surrounded by people who also yearned for something different.

With minimal digging on our creaky computer, I discovered that the school from *Bloomability* was a real place, perched on a Swiss hillside, sandwiched between snow-capped mountains and a palm tree–lined lake.

I brought it up to my parents one night over dinner.

At first, Mom and Dad seemed stunned into silence, genuinely confused about why I'd want to leave the loving bosom of our family, but they said they'd think about it.

Honestly, if anyone would say yes to sending their teenager across the world, it would be my parents. Mom wasn't like the other moms either, especially not the moms of Old Greenwich, Connecticut, whose motto, we joked, was Must Wear Pearls! The walls of her home office were packed with framed photos of her riding camels, standing in giant airplane engines, and sitting in the back of propeller planes, goggles perched on her head like a steampunk Amelia Earhart. One summer she registered the two of us for Arabic lessons, and later she moved to Syria for a month to practice the language and live with a host family. Mom had no intention of waiting for retirement to travel. She did all this with four children at home, refusing to let her identity of mother dictate the adventures she could or couldn't have. Mom was different, but she made it work. I could do the same, right?

I didn't have to wait long for their answer. One evening after Mom and Dad got home from their jobs in the city, they shed their coats and briefcases and suggested we have a chat in their bedroom. I trudged up the stairs after them, a sinkhole of dread forming in my stomach. Gingerly, I perched on the lumpy floral couch in their palatial room, Mom next to me, while Dad dragged an armchair closer to us both. After a beat, he cleared his throat and spoke, each word deliberate.

"Mom and I talked about your boarding school idea," he said. "We love that you want to travel like your mom. We considered it, but we both agreed the answer was no."

My mouth was already open to argue.

"Wait," he said, and held up his hand.

"We have another idea," Mom chimed in.

"We only have so many years with you in the house," Dad continued. "You're almost eighteen and we aren't willing to sacrifice a whole year with you."

In hindsight, of course, this is the sweetest thing I've ever heard, though I also understand that there was no way my parents could have afforded the $40,000 yearly tuition of the American School in Switzerland. We weren't *that* kind of Greenwich.

"How would you feel about going to Spain for a month?" asked Mom. "We could find a program for you to practice your Spanish."

Two of her six siblings were born in Puerto Rico, but Mom was the baby of her family and born after they'd settled in Miami. Her father rarely spoke Spanish to his children, for reasons unclear to us both. "If I could change one thing about my childhood," she later told me, "I would have learned to speak Spanish from infanthood. I have a bilingual family but was not bilingual. I am of a culture but not of a culture."

Enter my childhood's B story: a journey to native-level fluency and deeper connections to my family's heritage. The moment Mom learned she was pregnant with me, she hired a babysitter named Marta, who spoke only Spanish. Every year we visited Abuelo in Puerto Rico, and as soon as I could talk, I was my parents' unofficial translator. In middle school, when students were offered a choice between French and Spanish, I was in the front row of Señor Richard's advanced class, showing off my accent and trying to prove I wasn't just another gringa.

Even if I hadn't asked to attend some fancy Swiss boarding school, the Spain idea felt like it had been brewing all along. It wasn't a full year away from my life, but a month abroad was still plenty of time to reinvent myself.

"Oh my god, yes!" I shouted. "Yes, I definitely want to do that. Thank you!"

Dad nodded. "You're very welcome."

I can't remember how we found the program or anything else about my junior year, only that hope followed me down the echoing halls of Greenwich High School, books snug against my chest, looking out toward my own future instead of down through other people's stories.

THE SUMMER AFTER I turned seventeen, I took a red-eye to Madrid. The airport was hot, and I took off my madrigal choir sweatshirt and stuffed it into my bag as I weaved through yelling families, tourists, and frazzled airport staff. A family was ahead of me, walking fast, as a girl who appeared to be about five rushed behind them, little legs whirring as she struggled to keep up. She was holding a stuffed koala in one hand and dropped it without noticing. I reached down to pick it up. I hesitated for a millisecond as I calculated how to say the words to get Señor Koala back to his rightful owner.

"¡Perdòn!" I shouted, but they were already too far away. I was nervous about yelling in my not-yet-perfect Spanish inside an entire airport full of Spaniards, so I chased after them, dodging backpacks and slow-moving tourists. I reached the family as they turned toward baggage claim. I tapped the mother on the shoulder. "Perdòn."

She swung around. "¿Que?" she barked.

"Su hija," I panted. I couldn't remember the word for *dropped* so I held out the ratty koala.

"¡Gracias!" She gave the girl a side-eye and yelled something fast and harsh, but the girl didn't seem fazed. Meanwhile, I was beside myself with pride. I had basically given the Gettysburg Address in perfect Spanish. The woman hadn't switched to English, which meant my accent was flawless. The family moved on ahead, but I stood there beaming. This was the perfect decision. High school was so far away. Who cared if I wasn't invited to parties or had only one friend? While my peers were going to sailing camp or drinking beer in their basements, I was in *Spain*, alone, at seventeen. It didn't matter who I was back home; I saw a glimmer of what I was capable of and who I could become.

I wheeled my suitcase toward the exit, glancing at the welcome packet that told me where to meet the group. I heard shouting ahead, and even though the airport was noisy, this shouting stood out from the rest.

It was grating, nasal.

Americans.

I prayed and hoped it was a group of tourists, but the closer I got the more familiar it sounded. It was the sound of home—of teenagers yelling in an attempt to show the world that they're alive, they have friends, they leave their mark. I couldn't see them yet, but I knew what was coming. I looked for exit D and passed through the glass doors into the bright smoggy sunshine of Madrid. There, waiting by the curb, was a large bus with the words PATA STUDY ABROAD written in script on the side.

In a pulsing mass next to the bus were about twenty kids my age. In my memory, they resemble characters in a campy eighties movie—at least half of them wore visors, while the other half had double-popped collars in shades of pastel and sunglasses perched backward on their necks. The boys were all six feet tall with rumpled sandy hair. The girls were polished and grown-up looking with dark eyeliner and Tiffany bracelets shimmering on their wrists as they swept their hair from one shoulder to the other. In reality, of course, they were a mismatched group of awkward high school kids, but at that time in my life I couldn't see past my own differences to acknowledge anyone else's.

I slowed and touched my messy bun, hit with that well-worn feeling of social confusion and sensory overload. A tall man with close-cropped hair and a wide face not unlike Javier Bardem's was laughing with the kids when he caught my eye.

"Hello!" he said with a heavy accent. I stepped toward him, and the entire group looked at me. My cheeks hurt from smiling. Was I doing this right?

The circle parted, and the man said, "You must be Marian?"

"Yes, I am, hi!" My pitch was over-the-top chipper. Was I too loud?

"Estupendo." He made a note on his clipboard. "You are nearly our last one. Place your luggage under the bus and we will wait for our final student. Then you can introduce yourself."

I hovered next to the gaping luggage compartment, waiting for an opening to say who I was and where I was from.

One kid, a scrawny blond boy even shorter than me, didn't seem as engaged as the others. He gave me a little smile.

"Hi, I'm Clay," he said.

"Marian."

"I heard. Where are you from?"

"Connecticut," I said.

"Oh wow. I thought this was a Texas group."

"What do you mean?"

"Most of us are from San Antonio and Austin. This program's connected to our high school."

"Wait, what?"

"The PATA program? It's based in Texas. Most of the kids here know each other."

You have to be kidding me.

I'd assumed everyone would be traveling alone too. My throat tightened and my face fell and I could feel Bitch Marian reappear from where I'd left her. The moment of freedom in the airport was gone and I was back in high school, transplanted by crane to another country. How could I have thought I would be a completely different person after a six-hour flight?

Eventually, we piled onto the bus, and I took an empty row near the front, right behind Diego, our resident adult, who turned around to look at me, his right arm resting on the back of the seat.

"Are you okay?" he asked.

Any time I've braved a party or event, someone inevitably asks me this question. Something about my face or my body language or my placement in the room—usually in a corner with the safety of walls around me and a clear view—is a neon floodlight pulsing around my body. I know this question is meant with good intentions, but all it does is point out the obvious: I look so out of place, so different from everyone else, that it's cause for concern. And what am I supposed to say? No, I'm *not* okay? That I pinned all my hopes on this trip, but it turns out everyone is the same everywhere and I am the same everywhere and now I'm stuck here for a month? What would Diego even do with that information?

"I'm fine," I said tightly. "Jet lag."

"It is a bitch, yes?" Ah, he's a cool adult.

Diego tried to make conversation during the drive to Segovia, but he gave up after a few minutes when I didn't give anything back. I never quite get the rhythm of conversation right, the natural push and pull: I talk either way too much or not at all. With the right person, I'm willing to answer questions, but after I've done that and silence falls, I'm never sure what else to say. I didn't particularly care where he was from or how long he'd been in this job or what his favorite part of Spain was, so I stared quietly out the window, watching the urban landscape of Madrid pulsing around us, then the plains of Old Castile, with verdant mountains beyond, dense with pine and beech and juniper.

After our overnight stop in Segovia, where I wrote three full pages in my journal about the history of the Roman aqueducts, whose 167 arches were built without mortar, we hopped back on the bus and drove to Santander, a coastal town on a peninsula at the very northern tip of Spain, where we'd live with host families and attend classes at the local university.

We disembarked at a small plaza, where a smattering of adults waited to escort us to our new homes. I was paired with a room-mate named Natalie, a tall brunette from Austin, who wasn't part of the Texas high school either. Together we heaved our suitcases over the cobblestones and to our apartment, where an older woman opened the door and gave us a half smile before turning right around and walking up the stairs. Natalie and I glanced quickly at each other and stifled smiles. We twisted and turned, wrangling our suitcases up the narrow staircase. It took at least five minutes for us to reach the top, where our host mom, Carmen, waited on the landing.

Carmen let us into her apartment, which was small and cozy, with mauve walls and a bright galley kitchen. She showed us to a small room just off the foyer with matching twin beds covered with pale-blue comforters. It was a wonder how much else she'd managed to cram into the room: a stuffed monkey, a husband-and-wife teddy bear set, a collection of children's books I didn't recognize, framed pictures of her grown daughters, manicure supplies, and, on the walls, a collection of shelves hung at odd heights stuffed with knick-knacks. On the narrow nightstand wedged between our two beds, she'd placed a small white vase, which held a single faux rose.

"Para vosotros," she said, gesturing. *For you.*

As we unpacked, Natalie and I got to know each other. She was charming and kind and gasped when I said I wasn't from Texas.

"Oh, you don't know anyone!" she said. "That's terrible!" She didn't know anyone either, but I'd seen her chatting and laughing with the other kids in the back of the bus. She invited me to join them at a bar that night.

I'd had beer before, and champagne at family events, but never more than a small glass. I didn't like the way alcohol made me feel, and I hated the way it made other people act—messy and unpredictable. But wasn't I here to be free? To be different? But oh god I was so tired. A full day of traveling and hours on the bus. I looked longingly at my new bed.

"Please?" she said, noticing my hesitation. "It won't be fun without you!"

I pressed my lips together to hide a smile. I'd do anything for a compliment, especially one that made me feel wanted. "Sure." I shrugged.

After dinner—thinly sliced potatoes cooked into an omelet—Natalie and I changed before heading across the plaza to a bar that was, hilariously, Irish. Inside, the bass leaped down my throat like a demon looking for a host. The pulsing noise vibrated in my chest, my teeth. Sitting at the bar were a couple of the six-footers, including Drew, who had a mop of curly hair like Hugh Grant and a party trick that included popping out his front tooth, which he'd lost in a fight or a football game. Two girls, Peggy-Sue and Hailey, were perched on stools like flamingos. Hailey was perky with a blinding smile, and there was nowhere else she could be from than Texas. Her hair was bleached blond, and she was adorned with so much silver jewelry I worried for her safety. Peggy-Sue was the shape of an apple with hair nearly identical to Drew's but forced into a halo of gelled ringlets. They both had big smiles and immediately made space for me. A shot of bright-green liquid appeared, and I knocked it back. It tasted like licorice and I grimaced, but it warmed my belly, and the space around me softened. I turned to Natalie and Hailey and Peggy-Sue and Drew and Other Guy I Can't Remember, and I smiled and laughed, as brash and boisterous as the rest of them.

Here's the contradictory thing about my personality. When the winds are right, I can be extremely charming. My personality morphs from a pinprick to huge to a pinprick in seconds, like a fun house mirror. So for nearly an hour, I managed to put on a show, laughing and flirting and teasing, talking about nothing, but then the Texans got drunker and I got lonelier and the bar got louder and *click*. I powered down. My eyes glazed and my mouth slackened and words became impossible to form. I didn't yet understand that when this happens, I'm allowed to leave, so I stayed and I stayed and I stayed. Someone asked me what was wrong. The circle closed beyond me, and I inched behind Natalie like a barnacle.

Around midnight, my body was in so much physical pain I was practically moaning. I didn't care what the Texans thought anymore; I wanted my soft bed with the pale-blue duvet and the newlywed teddy bears, so I whispered to Natalie that I was too jetlagged to stay and teetered back to the apartment, climbed the four flights of stairs, and crawled into bed, sadder and lonelier than I had ever been.

THE FIRST FEW DAYS passed in a sea of self-pity. In hindsight, the other kids were probably funny and smart and adventurous, and the fact that they were in Spain at all meant we shared a common desire to see the world, but I didn't look hard enough to find it.

One afternoon, I was walking through the center of town alone, back to Carmen's mauve apartment, when I heard the rowdy laughter of Americans spilling out of a wine bar. Through the bar's enormous picture window, I spotted a few kids from my group laughing and drinking around a table, three pitchers of sangria between them. My plan to go back to Carmen's to chat over un cafecito and a Maria cookie seemed pathetic. I preferred to hang out with an old lady and practice my grammar than sit in a wine bar pretending to laugh with a bunch of Texan teens, but I couldn't help feeling like I *should* have wanted the latter.

At that exact moment María José, the program director, crossed the street in front of me and waved.

"Buenos días, Marian!" she called, stopping in front of me.

"Buenos días." I paused. Had a thought. Switched to English. "Um . . . could I talk to you for a second?"

She tilted her head and squinted. "Yes, of course." After nearly a week hearing her speak Spanish, I was surprised to watch her whole demeanor change when she spoke English. She sounded more tentative, seemed less of an authority figure. I waved her away from the bar to the windowless corner of the building. I glanced around to see if anyone could see us, then looked at my feet. My flip-flops were worn at the heels.

"The thing is—I thought this was a cultural exchange," I said, my tone hinting at more confidence than I felt. "Like, we'd all be learning Spanish and exploring Spain together."

"It *is* a cultural exchange."

"Well . . ." I hesitated, trying to find the words. "It feels more like a drinking program for teenagers."

"A *drinking* program?" I looked up at her then, and her eyebrows were practically swallowed by her hairline. I'd come this far, so it all spilled out of me.

"We've been here a week and every night they go out drinking and I just feel . . . that's not what I want to do."

"The other students are pressuring you to drink?"

"No, it's not that. I just expected we'd all be doing other things . . . together. This isn't why I came."

"No, of course not." She tapped her finger against her lips and said, "Let me handle this."

Of course, she knew what American teenagers would do while unattended in Europe, but she acted surprised and thoughtful and didn't make me feel like a tattletale, even though that's exactly what I was.

The next morning in class, the other kids were subdued. María José had written an email to our families, letting them know we'd been "drinking to excess" and "not reflecting the spirit of the program." Everyone got in trouble with their parents. Mom and Dad asked if I wanted to come home early.

I considered it. "The narc" was all anyone could talk about, though they never guessed it was me. For a week, they trudged back to their host families after class to practice grammar with old ladies and wander through the bustling ancient market that smelled like cured meats, and I felt all at once unchained from the pressure to pretend to live like them—and maybe a little smug that they were being forced to live like me. I didn't want to go home. I had a sort of guilty hope. A pinprick of magic called to me—not from the other kids, but Spain herself. For whatever reason, I knew I was supposed to stay and learn whatever she had to teach me.

I DIDN'T SPEND THE entire trip alone, but I have no memory of getting from point A to point B—from tattling to María José to sitting on the docks with Clay and Hailey, talking for hours while we watched the sunset. One day I was trying to ruin the entire group's trip and the next I was lying topless on the beach with Natalie, trying to mimic the thin and glossy Spanish women who chatted casually with their breasts out.

My memories toggle between joy and overwhelm. I remember ordering scoops of gelato every night after class and screaming with laughter at the Spanish word for hazelnut: *avellana*. To me, it sounded like *vagina*, and even though I hate hazelnut I ordered it just to be a clown.

I remember going to a bullfight and fleeing halfway through the first round to hide under the stands until it was over. Watching a bull get stabbed to death while thousands of people cheered flooded me with so much nausea I couldn't speak for the rest of the day.

I remember sitting on the curb of the plaza and kissing scrawny Clay, even though I had a boyfriend back home, because Clay had an obvious crush on me and it felt good to be wanted.

I remember, one day, when everyone retreated home after class to nap because they'd been out drinking the night before (they quickly found bars farther afield in which to drink in secret), but I was clear-headed and alive, so I took myself on a walk. I strolled through the familiar plaza and down a narrow cobblestoned alley. The buildings were all that burnt-orange color you rarely see in the States, giving the entire memory a sepia filter. A group of young boys was playing soccer in the square, and their ball came flying toward me. I caught it with a satisfying *thwack* and sent it sailing back. They shouted their thanks and I joked that they should kick better next time. A few minutes later, a woman approached me and asked for the time, which I gave to her fluidly and without hesitation. When I was alone, no one spoke to me in English. On the streets of Santander, I was someone else entirely. I belonged here.

I practically skipped to the beach, where the sand was gold and the water clear. It was peak travel season and a swell of tourists surged around me. In the chaos of the unknown, alone in this city, I was, somehow, calm. I didn't need another person to enjoy this moment. In fact, the moment was better because no one's energy was buzzing in my ear, distracting me from how much joy there was to witness in the world.

Down the main thoroughfare along the beach, I spotted a friendly café, where I ducked in to order my new favorite meal: un sandwich mixto y un café con leche. A thrill moved through my stomach as I spoke to the waiter. I sat alone at a table outside and inhaled the salty air, the fresh coffee. The waves lapped against sailboats and retaining walls. Tourists shouted. A busker was playing rapid guitar and the music rode toward me on the breeze.

I had become Dinnie—grown-up, adventurous, and woven into a tapestry more vibrant than my previously muted world. I had become *every* character in my books, and for the first time my aloneness felt like freedom.

—7—

Copycat

HER NAME CAME TO ME IN THE MAIL. *AMÉLIE ADAMO.* I'D NEVER HEARD
a more sensational name in my life, and she would be *my* roommate
at a school I'd stumbled upon mostly by chance—a small liberal arts
college in Davidson, North Carolina, called, conveniently, Davidson.

Davidson's roommate assignment process was the stuff of leg-
end. Before registration, we filled out lengthy surveys, including
a personality test and a housing preference form. The admissions
staff bragged about Davidson weddings and Davidson godparents.
Nearly half the students chose to bunk with their freshman-year
roommates all four years of school, so when I got my match, I was
filled with romantic ideas that Amélie wouldn't just be the girl with
whom I split a futon but the highs and lows of my life.

But god, her name. It was the kind of name people don't have
in real life, the kind of name you say twice for emphasis, like James
Bond: Amélie, Amélie *Adamo.*

But it was real, and so was she.

We talked on the phone once before school started. I'd climbed
into my car after a long day at my summer job packing boxes for
a meditation music distributor, when my phone rang and an unfa-

miliar voice—high-pitched and airy—came through the other end. I can't remember what we talked about, but I do remember hanging up with a balloon in my chest.

She's kind, I thought. *This could be great.*

Everything I knew about female friendships I learned from *The Baby-Sitters Club* and *The Sisterhood of the Traveling Pants*. When teen girls make friends, you do everything together: you hug in the halls before and after class, you share lip gloss and tampons and clothes. You know each other's deepest, darkest secrets. Boyfriends come and go, but girlfriends are forever.

I'd had a few friendships over the years, but they'd all fizzled out, leaving me friendly enough with a few people, but never truly connected with any one person. At lunch I'd sit with Margot and the theater kids, and after school I'd sometimes walk next door to Dave's house to watch him and his buddies play video games, but I didn't *belong* to any of them.

The thing I wanted more than anything else was a permanent place in a tight-knit group of girlfriends, and everyone told me college was how I'd get there.

THE DRIVE TO NORTH Carolina was thirteen hours, and my stomach clenched when we turned off exit 30 and into the small, leafy suburb of Davidson. Dad sniffed from the driver's seat, then dabbed his eyes, but mine were locked on the town, with its brick sidewalks flanked by local shops with charming stone flowerpots and fluttering American flags out front.

Just east of Main Street, a manicured lawn lolled toward a collegiate building four stories tall with a domed roof and stately columns. It was nearly autumn, but we were farther south than I'd ever been, and it didn't smell like leaves or wet earth but sunbaked stone, grass, and something sweet and floral. My seat belt was already unbuckled by the time Dad came to a complete stop in the parking lot. Class didn't start for a few days, but the paths teemed with students, the freshmen obvious with their darting eyes and platoons of parents.

Something caught my eye on the brick sidewalk. Hundreds of green-and-black splotches were smeared every few inches, like gum on the streets of Manhattan, almost pressed into the stone itself. I'd later learn they were the bodies of cankerworms, and their gooey corpses littered campus for weeks every year, following us to our rooms, hitching rides on the bottom of our shoes.

My dorm was a squat brick building, the first in a row under the canopy of mature willow oaks. I looked for Amélie among the crowd outside the residence hall, wondering whether I'd recognize her from her Facebook profile photo. A tall sporty redhead met my eye, but I looked away and fumbled for my key card before realizing I should have smiled.

I was the first to arrive at Little #310, the beds still bare and vacuum tracks showing in the gray carpet, the window left open to encourage a breeze. I left my suitcase by the door, sat on the bed in the farthest corner, and bounced once to test its comfort.

"Marian?" I heard a high voice behind me and turned. It was her.

She was smaller in real life, tiny like a fairy, with dark blond hair and long bangs that swooped over her forehead. She wore jean shorts and a simple brown T-shirt.

"Amélie!" I shouted.

"Call me Ami." She smiled and glanced down at my suitcase that blocked her way into the room.

I apologized and rushed forward to roll it out of her way.

"Oh, it's okay!" She waved me off and rewarded me with another luminous smile. Behind her, a tall blond man and a short dark-haired woman appeared. Before I could introduce myself, my parents pushed their way forward.

"Jim," said Dad, jutting out his hand.

"George," the man said back.

The mothers smiled while Ami and I stood by the door. Our parents were now asking each other how the drive was and where they got breakfast that morning and what part of Ohio they were from, before eventually wearing themselves out and leaving us behind with lingering, tearful goodbyes.

Ami and I stood facing each other in this strange room in a hall full of strange girls. I had no idea what to say. Ami's eyes darted toward the bustling, fluorescent hall, and she played with the loose threads on her shorts.

The endless silence pressed in on my ears, so I laughed in a sharp bark and shouted, "Well, THIS is super awkward!"

Oh no, what the hell is wrong with me? What an insane thing to say. She's going to hand in her roommate reassignment paperwork tonight if I don't get my shit together. I covered my nose with my hand and flared my nostrils as wide as they would go.

"SO AWKWARD!" she burst out with a laugh. That laugh made my whole body tingle.

"It's like . . . hi, I live with you now," I continued, encouraged. "Hope we don't hate each other!"

"Hope you don't smell like old cheese and hover at my bedside watching me sleep," she countered.

We skipped the small talk and jumped straight into friendly teasing as we unpacked our clothes and posters and relics from home.

Our dorm orientation was in an hour and I nervously asked, "Do you want to go together?"

"Please!" she said. "You're the only person I know. Don't leave me!"

I grinned so hard my face hurt. *She likes me! She wants to be near me too!*

On our first day of class, we were walking together down Main Street to grab coffee when a man in a rusty pickup slowed down beside us and drawled, "Nice ass, ladies!"

Without even pausing to hesitate I shouted, "SHUT THE FUCK UP, PERVERT." I was loud enough to hurt both our ears, but I'm not sure he heard me over the roar of his engine.

I froze, knowing *this* would be the thing that scared her—my complete lack of filter, my predilection toward harshness, anger, rage. I turned to her and grimaced, apologetic before she said a word.

"You're the best," she said and looped her arm through mine.

There it was: a symbol of real live female friendship. I could see us from the outside, girlfriends from the movies, laughing and linked arm in arm. I tried not to clutch her too tightly.

We stuck together during those first few days at Davidson, until eventually that's how we moved through the world, one of us never far from the other. She was the funniest person I'd ever met, and I was her enraptured audience. We'd exercise around the campus track cracking jokes, wheezing with laughter until we couldn't stand upright, never mind run. Ami was the first person I could be my full self around. Any time I said something that would normally have made someone else pull away, Ami drew closer. When I tentatively admitted that I didn't like to party or drink and was worried that I'd miss out on the College Experience, she gasped. "Me too! I want to be in bed at nine with a book." Which is what we did most evenings, climbing into our lofted beds, never falling asleep without whispering good night.

In no time at all, Ami had filled in me the need to belong. In return, I found a need that I could fill for her.

It happened one day in the cafeteria when we sat next to the soccer team at a long table by the windows. Ami was wearing a T-shirt that read HERE COMES THE SUN in kitschy seventies bubble print. Nate, the sandy-haired captain of the soccer team, swooped in on her as soon as we'd settled in with our trays.

"What does your shirt say?" he asked, squinting at her chest.

Ami, oblivious, said, "Oh, it says—"

"No, I can't see it," he interrupted. He mimed pulling his own shirt down, and without realizing what he was trying to do, Ami did the same, pulling her T-shirt tight over her breasts so he could "see the words."

"What the fuck are you doing, Nate?" I snapped. "Leave her alone."

Ami glanced at me, eyebrows raised, and I gave my head a small shake. I'd explain it to her later.

"You're no fun," he pouted.

"Yeah, and you're gross."

I spoke up for her when she couldn't. I accompanied her to the bank to open her first-ever account and I yelled at catcallers and idiotic basketball players. I became her protector. For me, she issued invitations when she went out, introduced me to her theater friends, and let me borrow from her extensive DVD collection. It was like falling in love, but better.

Ami was more like me than any person I'd ever met, except for one thing, and that difference was everything. Everyone else loved her too.

Around our second week, a few girls stopped by our room and greeted Ami by name. I still hadn't met anyone yet. Whenever I left for class, I scurried through campus with my head down, too anxious to look up, knowing I'd probably tell an inappropriate joke if required to make small talk.

Ami was draped against the doorframe and giggling, while I lurked behind her, unsure what to do with my hands. I walked over to the futon and straightened the pillows. I opened my laptop and pretended to check something. Then I walked to the sink—maybe there was a dish I could wash? I paced the room, eavesdropping on their conversation, waiting for an opportunity to jump in.

They aren't here for you.

But did I look rude just standing there? Shouldn't I introduce myself?

Ami made it look so easy. She laughed with a loud HA-HA-HA, but it was bright and irresistible. Her posture was casual, comfortable.

"Can you *believe* what Valentina said in class today?" Ami faux-whispered.

"Oh god, I know. It's like, could she be any more obvious?" said the brunette who'd come to visit. She had eyelashes so long she looked like Cindy-Lou from Whoville.

I had no idea what they were talking about, but clearly Ami had made good enough friends that they knew where we lived and would drop by to gossip. I couldn't name a single person from my classes. It dawned on me then: as incredible as Ami was and as lucky as I was to have her, this one difference between us was enormous.

I couldn't figure out if I wanted her to myself, or if I simply wanted to be her.

WHEN FALL DESCENDED AND the air turned crisp and earthy, Ami grabbed a brown bomber jacket from her closet. She pulled it on across her slender shoulders and zipped it up. It had an enormous fur hood, oversize decorative buttons, and a thick waistband that rode up her narrow hips. It was the coolest thing I'd ever seen.

"Oh my god, your *coat*," I gasped.

"Thank you!" she said, petting the fur like it was a small animal. "Abercrombie."

I filed that knowledge away, and for all of November and December, I had that jacket tab saved on my browser and agonized over whether I should pull the trigger. First, it was expensive, and I was broke. Second, I couldn't buy a coat she had, could I?

But every time she wore it, she looked so effortlessly pulled together. The definition of cool. That jacket was everything that made Ami the popular one and me, jacketless, the dark shadow friend. If I looked more like Ami, maybe people would gravitate toward me too.

In middle school it had been cute to wear the same clothes as your friends. Chelsea, Elena, and I had matching "best friend" necklaces, and once, Elena and I attended a bowling birthday party wearing the same gray pants and red T-shirt. Wasn't that the real definition of friendship—sameness? In *The Sisterhood of the Traveling Pants*, author Ann Brashares wrote, "Sometimes it seems like we're so close we form one single complete person rather than four separate ones." If a pair of miraculously well-fitting jeans could bring good luck to four friends, maybe a cool jacket could impart some of Ami's lovability to me.

I was also deeply insecure about the way I looked. I felt completely incapable of dressing myself or looking the part of other teenagers. One day during my senior year of high school, I dressed in a new outfit I'd bought at the Stamford mall—brown high-heeled boots, a corduroy knee-length skirt, and a striped turtleneck. I walked through the long hall of Greenwich High with a satisfying clacking that made me feel tall and imposing and put together, until a senior shouted, "Hola, Señora Tierra!" and I realized I looked exactly like our forty-year-old Spanish teacher and not at all like Lexi, the queen popular girl whose style I envied, with her silky sheet of blond hair, ripped jean skirt, and unscuffed Uggs.

I couldn't riff; I could only copy.

When Ami and I left Davidson for winter break that year, promising to Skype on Christmas Day, I found an identical Abercrombie coat on eBay for only thirty dollars. I didn't hesitate for a second before clicking Buy Now. I waited for its delivery every day, and when it arrived on the front stoop of my parents' house, I sliced the package open and pulled on the coat in one smooth motion.

I looked amazing. It flattered my figure; it was warm; I was cool. I paraded around Old Greenwich that week knowing I at least *looked* like a real girl. I just needed to figure out what I'd say to Ami when we got back on campus.

When we arrived back at Davidson that January, Ami and I were unpacking in our room when I eased the coat from my suitcase.

"Look what my parents got me for Christmas!" I lied.

"No way!" she said, excited. "Now we can be twins." I can still feel the thrill of my relief. She was so good. So kind.

The jacket, of course, was the first in a long line of attempts to capture the magic of Ami.

In April, she bought a sugary-sweet perfume from Urban Outfitters that smelled like spring and sunshine. I rarely wore perfume, and when I did it was musky and deep. I owned one bottle—matte black with a hipster drawing of a gun on the front. My instincts always led toward dark and brooding.

After Ami left for class one morning, I opened her closet door and spritzed a little of that perfume on myself. I left for class in a waft of her, and for a moment I was sunshine too.

I passed her in a stairwell later that day and she shouted down, "Hey! You smell like Spun Sugar!"

I quickly lied, saying I had a sample of that same perfume from a magazine. I'm not sure she believed me.

The next month, Ami and her new friend Layla went shopping at Birkdale Village near campus and came home with matching knit hats. I seethed with jealously and immediately bought one in a different color. I didn't even lie this time; I just said I wanted to be part of the group. Ami nodded thoughtfully and said we should all wear them that night when we walked to dinner.

Ami and I shared a room our sophomore year too; we didn't even discuss it. We were best friends and we lived well together. I'm not sure she knew that underneath my love was pain and jealousy. One long weekend, Ami visited her parents back in Ohio while I stayed on campus. After a day luxuriating in my aloneness, I got an idea. Ami had bought a pair of teal knee-length boots that I coveted. I knew my copying was becoming excessive, and there would eventually be an end to Ami's understanding, so I had no intention of buying those boots for myself. But she wasn't here, was she? And her clothes were just sitting there, alone and unworn.

I opened her closet with a creak and examined the treasures

within. It was as if all of Ami were laid out before me, and I could reach out and pluck out her eyes and her hair and her skin and patch it on myself like a desperate Frankenstein.

I pulled on the boots and, figuring I might as well run the full mile, her flowy blue Free People dress too. Then I headed out the door and into the bright North Carolina day with nowhere to go, strutting around pretending to be Ami, as if her clothes would rub her essence off on me.

They didn't. I kept waiting to get caught, for her to jump out of the bushes and cry, "You're a freak!"

I was still me, dour and surly, and she was still a delicate bubble floating above. Instead of embracing the impulses that made me unique, my brain could see only one acceptable version of what it meant to be a college girl. There was no room for any other type of woman, never mind a serious, autistic one. Everyone loved Ami; people tolerated me. The longer our friendship continued, the more I doubted she liked me at all. How could she? I was a mangy barking shelter dog nipping at her heels, following her around campus, begging for scraps. I stole her clothes and latched myself onto her friends. As the months passed, I braced myself to be dumped. Why did she even like me? When was she going to leave? This couldn't last forever.

I had to know what she was thinking.

AMI WROTE DAILY IN her sparkly red journal. I would see it lying there on her desk, so innocuous and small, but I knew, without even opening it, that inside it was huge. It was the whole world.

I don't know what I expected to find that winter afternoon, but I stared at her diary for a long time, at war with myself about whether to open it. I eventually justified it with this: *Reading her diary will help me be a better friend.* If I knew how Ami's mind worked, I had a better chance of understanding how *people* worked. If I knew what she didn't like about me, I could change it.

The logic was simple, but it nauseated me too. The idea that any friend had thoughts about me they wouldn't share brought me right back to that fourth-grade day in the closet. I had quickly learned that people who claimed to like me couldn't be trusted, because underneath the surface was a simmering litany of complaints—and since I couldn't tell when someone was upset with me, I must always be on guard.

With a rippling of terror, I cracked open Ami's diary.

Inside were many things I already knew—stories and anxieties and hopes and dreams we talked about late into the night: Her crush on a guy in the theater department who looked like a very tall squirrel and absolutely did not deserve her. Her classes and grades and a role she desperately wanted in an experimental play about a parrot.

And me.

I spotted my name in a short entry about how I kept calling her a slut. It was the early 2000s and girls called each other *whore* and *bitch* and *slut* as a greeting. On campus I'd see two friends walking toward each other and one would wave and smile and the other would shout, "Hey, slut!" and they'd laugh and walk together to class. I saw that this was how women talked to each other, so I mirrored it back to Ami. When she walked into our room, arms weighed with books, I'd look up from my whirring Dell and cheerfully yell, "Hey, slut!"

I remember nothing about her facial expression, only that I said it, and now I knew it bothered her. With relief, I thought, *Okay, I can change this.* It felt like ticking a box on a long checklist toward normalcy. One down, unknown to go. I vowed to immediately stop the name-calling and reverted back to our pet name for each other: Muffin. Our freshman year, I accidentally called her Muffin, which was the nickname I'd given our family dog, whom I adored. Mock-offended, Ami called me Muffin back, and the rest is history. She's still in my phone as Muffin Adamo.

I didn't read any more of her diary that night, but once I got a glimpse inside the inner workings of the girl I wanted to please and understand and be, I couldn't stop myself from coming back. I couldn't read her, but I could read her diary. It was the relationship manual I had desperately craved.

Weeks later, I read this:

I've asked her so many times, but Marian gets into bed by stepping on the rungs of my bed and it wakes me up. She keeps doing it. I can't sleep!

I remembered Ami asking me about this, but I kept forgetting. Reading it on the page was like a warning letter from the IRS. I never forgot again.

Another day she wrote, *Marian is so fake.*

At the time, I didn't understand what she meant, and I kind of skipped over this feedback, but clearly some part of my brain filed this away because the word still haunts me.

Fake.

Of course I was fake. My friendships only worked because I reflected people back to themselves. I mirrored mannerisms and outfits. By the time I was nineteen I had been called *lazy, moody, sensitive, harsh, weird, annoying, mean,* and *buzzkill* by everyone from my parents to my teachers to my most beloved friends. Of course I flattened myself into the purest, shiniest mirror I could, focusing all my energy into matching their every movement like those icebreaker games we played in school.

Katherine May, author of *The Electricity of Every Living Thing*, learned she was autistic in her late thirties, but she'd been pretending to be someone else long before then. She wrote, "I learned to ask after people's children from a woman on a train. I learned to crack self-effacing jokes from a colleague who always got away with murder. I was a parrot, a mynah bird, and even if I were able to, I wasn't willing to turn it all off just to convince others of my need for care."

Every autistic woman I've spoken with or whose work I've read has a story about their copycat tendencies. Some carried physical scripts so they'd know exactly what to say and when. Sometimes these scripts came from movies; others were transcribed conversations they kept tucked in their notebooks to reference later.

Neurodiversity and mental health advocate Mara McLoughlin told me a story about her attempts to fit in during elementary school. In fifth grade, Mara decided life would be better if she became her cousin. She hatched a plan to dye her hair, wear colored contacts, and speak in a southern accent. "If I wasn't myself," she said, "then the other kids would like me."

Another woman I spoke with said that she has set personalities for each social group, and for years never realized how often she switched between them. She'd be in her high school hallway chatting to a friend in one specific way, but if a different friend walked over to join them, she'd switch midstory into that friend's personality, making group dynamics nearly impossible, like trying to maintain a single conversation in six languages at once.

For me, it's like a game of Guess Who. Inside my brain is a plastic flip board of all the different women I've met through the years. When I'm with the brilliant poet who talks in puns and rarely smiles, and with people like her, I'll rack my brain for an opinion on the latest adaptation of *Pride and Prejudice* (which I've never read) or political figures (whose names I never bother to learn). With the sporty hiker who always has weekend plans, I'll quash my desire to talk for twenty minutes about my latest video game and instead mention a hike I took ten years ago. Within five seconds I can flip over their card and transform myself into the type of woman I believe each expects me to be. If I draw a blank, I'll whip out my performance of the over-the-top loud, funny, charming, say-anything Marian to smother the quiet, brooding woman who lives underneath.

In the autistic community, this behavior is called *masking*. Masking is the act of suppressing your natural instincts and replacing them with learned, often rehearsed behaviors so you can fit in. Which makes sense now, looking back on those months I spent wearing Ami's clothes and reading her journal.

The last entry I read was a few months after I started. It had gotten to a point that every time I saw her writing, my heart would split wide open and the whole room would cave in around me. *She's writing about me*, I'd think. I couldn't focus on anything until she left the room and I could fling open the book to learn about myself.

I think Marian's been reading my diary. So what if she has?

In hindsight, I must have been so obvious. I'd immediately stopped calling Ami insulting names. I'd stopped using her bed as a ladder. I stopped reading her journal then too.

Before my diagnosis, when I thought about this period of my life, I was filled with so much shame that I could only skirt over the memory like a tender bruise. I wanted to crawl in a hole and die just thinking about having worn her clothes like some Talented Mr. Ripley or having eavesdropped on her most personal, private thoughts that were never meant for anyone's eyes, let alone mine.

Hearing stories from other autistic women has helped me forgive college Marian for all the ways she tried to mend her brokenness. I didn't trust myself to be interesting or lovable on my own. I assumed the things that made a person worthy were external, like blue boots and sugary perfume or the number of people who stopped by my dorm room after class.

For some autistics, masking works. It allows us to belong to a community, which is apparently our most ancient impulse. From Psychology 101 to self-help books, we hear one message more than any other: Humans are social creatures. We're not meant to go through life alone. One article I read in *Psychology Today* said it best—our social network is "the most profound predictor of our health and well-being."

But what if friendship isn't your natural instinct?

What if, no matter how hard you try, people just don't like the real you?

— 8 —

Lazy Failure Slob

I DIDN'T FAIL OUT OF SCHOOL, BUT I CAME CLOSE. IT STARTED SLOWLY, imperceptibly, after the newness of college had worn off, a few months into my freshman year.

At 7 a.m., I fumbled to snooze the metallic music blaring from my Motorola Razr. My bed was right next to the window, and the sun streamed into my blurry eyes. I covered my face with my hands. I was being pulled back into the erasure of sleep, weightless and dark. Every few seconds my body twitched, as if my mind were trying to jolt me back to life. I had class in an hour. I had to get up. I had to climb down the ladder of my lofted bed and creep out the door so as not to wake Ami, who was smart enough not to register for 8 a.m. classes. I had to brush my teeth and wash my face in the echoey hall bathroom, the water running down my arms and splattering all over the sink and floor. Then I'd have to spread thick globs of benzoyl peroxide slowly and gently across my acne-covered skin.

"You need to be gentler with your face," Ami told me once, while teaching me a new skin-care method she'd discovered, and so this task always felt excruciatingly slow, like I was wasting years of my life standing in front of the mirror with a face shiny like a blobfish. The gooey mess took forever to dry, and for five, ten, fifteen minutes

I'd pace our room on tiptoes, fanning my face, itching to wipe it all off while deliberating over what to wear.

Getting dressed meant juggling two opposing forces: the need to select an outfit that would help me fit in while simultaneously avoiding the desire to rip my skin off.

Changing my clothing was one of the few ways I could feel like everybody else, but unless I had a specific outfit to copy, I would freeze, facing my mismatched wardrobe of styles I could never seem to pull together—airy dresses from Urban Outfitters, pilling preppy sweaters from Old Navy, knockoff Birkenstocks from DSW. Everything I owned made me feel frumpy. In photos from that time, I look one step behind everyone else. While other Davidson girls wore bikinis to Lake Norman, I'd be in a blue empire-waisted dress. At parties, Ami's friends danced in slinky, strappy tops, while I wore a short-sleeved floral blouse with a ruffly collar. I couldn't quite figure out how to blend in, and it took every ounce of energy to get a quarter of the way there.

Then there was the comfort factor. A simple bra caused so much unpleasantness. Raising my hand in class would cause the underwire to shift a millimeter against my ribcage and the hairs on my body to stand up as if a ghost had moved through me, and I'd completely forget the question I'd meant to ask. While talking to a classmate, all my attention would fixate on the button of my jeans digging into my belly button or the caked layers of acne medication and lotion and makeup crusting on my face like a dirty sheet mask.

So no, I did not want to get out of bed and face the endless list of miserable chores that awaited me.

Once I'd gotten my alarm to stop harassing me from deep inside the covers, I mentally sorted through my closet. Unable to come up with anything that ticked all the boxes, my mind drifted to my upcoming class. Cognitive Psychology with Professor Doyle, the most frustrating human on the planet. He was a pencil of a man with a head of receding wispy blond hair. He talked and talked about the neural bases of mental processes, and I could never follow the thread of what he was saying. It'd loop in circles in the air and under our desks and out the window before coming back and landing in my lap with a whisper.

I spent hours on his assignments, writing essays about brain research methodology, only for them to come back with *D*'s scribbled on the front in red ink. Until this point, I'd thought I was smart—I had a 4.6 GPA in high school and prided myself on my work ethic and ability to focus for long stretches of time—but my grades kept sinking.

Religion in the Movies: C+
Renaissance Art in Europe: C−
Biology of Plants: C−
Intro to Hispanic Literature and Culture: C−

Thinking about Professor Doyle and my poor grades was enough for me to surrender to the duvet. With great relief I pulled the blankets over my head and plummeted back to sleep.

ONE AFTERNOON AMI AND I sat at our respective desks, trying to get through a mountain of homework. Mine was Spanish, a subject I could usually ace with my eyes closed and hands tied behind my back, but at Davidson, the more advanced grammar rules taunted me, barely visible and impossible to catch. It was as if I'd never spoken a word of Spanish in my life and had somehow been thrust into a college-level class by mistake. I stared at the assignment for fifteen minutes, but the page stayed blank.

My desk was tucked underneath our lofted beds, which hovered above me, beckoning. I closed my laptop and moaned into my hands. "I can't doooo this."

"Me too," said Ami, stretching.

"Will you judge me if I get into bed?" I asked. It was all I wanted in the whole world, but I feared her judgment more than my fatigue.

"NO!" She whipped around in her chair and smiled. "That is *literally* the only thing I want to do right now."

"Then let's do it." I stood, rubbing the indents from the backs of my thighs.

The sun was bright through the windows, and student laughter floated up to us. It felt obscene to even consider wasting this beautiful day, but we were giddy for it.

"You know, we could . . . watch a movie," Ami suggested.

She ran a finger along the glossy DVD cases stacked neatly on her desk. "I have *Garden State*, *I Love Lucy*, *Harry Potter*, *The O.C.* . . ."

I was overtaken by greed, dizzy and powerful. Growing up, my parents didn't allow TV, so I'd missed all the good teen shows—*Gilmore Girls*, *Buffy*, *Dawson's Creek*, and *The O.C.* I'd heard of Ryan and Marissa, Seth and Summer, as if they were seniors at my school whose lives we dissected with whispered reverence. I, however, was like a foreign exchange student constantly interjecting with "Wait, who?" and "What happened?" My lack of pop culture knowledge was such a part of my personhood that my college application essay was specifically about growing up without television. Occasionally I'd run into a teacher on campus who'd exclaim in awe, "Marian Schembari—you're the No-TV Girl!"

It had taken until this very moment to realize the freedom I now possessed.

"You know, I've never seen *The O.C.* . . ." I replied, trying not to seem too eager.

"I would totally watch it again," Ami said, pulling the slim case from the tidy stack. "It's soooo good."

Ami popped the DVD into the player. We'd put the TV on the top shelf of our closet, so the only real way to see it clearly was from up on our lofted beds. She sat in hers and I sat in mine, pillows propped behind my back and comforter folded around me like a cocoon. The weight of it pushed me into the mattress and the first tinny notes from the opening piano sequence filled the room. My shoulders dropped and my pulse slowed. I hadn't even realized I'd been panting. I was still and quiet, my brain completely turned off. For the next forty-five minutes, nobody needed anything from me; I was required to do nothing, go nowhere, be no one.

We watched the first two seasons that month, rushing back from class to crawl into bed and belt out the opening song together, "*Califooooornia, here we cooooome!*"

After that, we made our way through Ami's entire collection before discovering a new service called Netflix that sent DVDs to my Davidson PO box. By sophomore year, Ami and I had devoured all seven seasons of *Gilmore Girls* and moved on to *The L Word*.

In the beginning, I waited for her like one-half of a married couple, but Ami was social and busy with theater, so I often found myself alone in our room. Without supervision, I'd attend one class, then rush back home to catch every show I'd missed in high school. One long weekend while Ami was away, I watched forty-nine episodes of *Lost*. Unable to even make it up to my bed, I flung myself across the futon like old laundry and didn't move until Monday, surviving on Welch's white grape juice and Wheat Thins draped in Cheez Whiz.

Living at Davidson felt like being in an endless play with no intermission, trying so hard to look right, act right, say the right thing. The world was a stage, and my door was the curtain, a heavy veil that stripped away every last layer of my performance. The moment I passed through, my mask fell away and all that was left was oblivion.

GROWING UP, WE CALLED Mom the Energizer Bunny. On Sundays before church, while the boys and I stayed cozy in bed until the very last second, Mom was awake at 5 a.m. for her daily ten-mile run.

She came home, showered, blow-dried her hair, dressed, and put on makeup, then tidied the kitchen and had a hot breakfast ready by the time we poured out of our rooms and slid down the stairs like sentient slime.

Dad was her opposite, which makes me wonder whether her frustration at having a sullen, low-energy daughter was a spillover from having a husband who was the same. On weekends, she'd roll her eyes as he began his pilgrimage upstairs for an afternoon nap, calling behind him, "I'm going to rest my eyes for a few minutes."

"Don't be like your father," she would warn me. The worst thing you could do in our house was rest.

The problem was, I seemed to need so much of it.

Laziness was my secret shame. It attached itself to my skin during childhood and I lugged it with me to Davidson. Here I was, free at last, able to make choices for myself, but with an open day, I wouldn't choose to audition for a choir, or play Frisbee on the lawn, join a club, tutor at the local high school, or volunteer at a soup kitchen. It all felt so deeply and utterly *exhausting*. Without Mom chiding me to get some fresh air, I swung too hard in the opposite direction. I was lazy, exactly who she believed me to be.

NO MATTER HOW PERSISTENTLY I bullied myself, I did not magically wake up one morning with boundless energy and a zest for life. Instead, by senior year I stopped showering.

Hygiene had always felt like a never-ending burden rather than luxurious self-care, but the pressure to fit in outweighed my desire to forgo it. In college, during my fourth year of near-constant sensory overload and social anxiety, it transformed from an inconvenience to an impossibility.

The trickle of water down my forearms after I splashed water on my face was like ants crawling on my skin, and brushing my teeth was an insufferable monotony that also included the mild torture of the sharp and overwhelming taste of mint . . . and I had to do this twice a day, every day, forever until I died? *No fucking thank you.*

And don't get me started on showering. It is literally twelve thousand steps: How does anyone have time to do anything else?

Take this random Thursday afternoon in October: I was lying, cozy in bed, watching *Buffy*, my latest TV obsession. Around 8 p.m., I realized I should probably peel myself from under the comforter and take a shower. I'd had two classes that day, followed by a three-hour shift at the art gallery where I worked, followed by dinner with Ami and her friend Trevor, who'd told me over tacos that a bunch of his friends thought I was "terrifying." I'd collapsed into bed, a little teary, to disappear into the story of Buffy and Angel, whose romance rivaled any I'd ever had, whose friendships were kind and respectful, who honored each other's strengths. Why would I leave the safety of my room to talk to people I didn't understand or particularly care for, when every person I needed was right there on my laptop?

But bathing was an activity everyone else did daily, so that meant I had to take off my clothes, decide whether they were clean enough to wear again or if they would fit into my overflowing laundry basket. I had to walk to the bathroom and hope it wasn't in use. If it was, it was all over for that night; I'd shower tomorrow. If it was free, I'd have to get my whole body wet and remember all the parts that needed cleaning. Did I need to shave my legs? Wash my hair? Washing my naturally curly hair meant staying in the bathroom for an extra hour so I could dry and style it. "Naturally curly" is a cosmic joke, requiring special shampoo applied in a very specific way, followed by an enormous amount of sticky gel and careful, painstaking, mind-numbing diffusing. The thought of all those decisions, all those steps, plopped an anvil onto my chest, and I could no longer physically move.

What was the point? I only had one class the next day and didn't need to impress anyone. I'd spend the rest of the day in bed anyway. Why go through this charade of self-care? It wasn't for me, not really.

It was for everyone else. Truly caring for myself looked like talking to no one, lying in bed watching *Buffy*, and occasionally turning over to prevent bedsores.

Still, the internal voice, which sounded a lot like my mother, said, *For Heaven's sake, Marian, that's disgusting. NORMAL PEOPLE CLEAN THEMSELVES.*

I tuned her out by clicking Next Episode.

Every few days, I haphazardly rinsed and brushed and splashed. I stopped doing anything with my hair and defaulted to a crooked bun perched on top of my head. I stopped caring about my clothes and wore the same black yoga pants and ratty blue sweatshirt every day.

Nobody noticed or asked questions. Something inside me was capable enough, scared enough, motivated enough, to do *exactly* the bare minimum to appear not like the witch in a hovel I truly was but like a tired college student buried under mountains of homework and late-night frat parties. I managed *C*'s and *D*'s and occasional *B*'s, and I had enough friends (through Ami) who showered me with compliments about how "unique" I was. "I love how you just don't care," said one. "You're just so *yourself*!" said another.

I didn't want to be myself. I wanted to be them.

Once every week or two, I'd yell at myself loudly enough to get up, walk to the local coffee shop, and do my homework somewhere public. For an hour, it was lovely. Summit Coffee had a second floor full of lumpy mismatched couches, packed with students whose heads were bent over papers and laptops. Their energy made me feel part of campus life, if only for an afternoon.

I'm one of them. Even though I wasn't gossiping at a table full of people or working on a group project, and even though I couldn't greet the baristas by name, I'd left the house! I'd done something! My life had meaning again.

When I finished for the day and headed home, I crawled into bed to watch *Buffy*. I'd earned it. I'd done my bit.

The next day, when it came time to get up, I couldn't.

A few weeks passed before I guilted myself into going out again—this time to the library or a party. I could sustain a broad smile and itchy costume for an hour before turning to Ami and whispering, "I have to go."

"Yeah, let's blow this popsicle stand," she'd say.

She was the only person who never made me feel like a loser.

On one of those days, in a surprising burst of energy, I made an appointment with a school therapist, who was housed in a small beige room inside the student health building. I was aware that my behavior wasn't that of a vibrant, busy college student, and it didn't feel great to look at my friends with their theater auditions and extracurriculars and crushes and frat parties, knowing I could never touch any of it. Something appeared to be broken inside me, and I figured counseling might fix it. Davidson offered free therapy, so why not give it a shot?

"I feel like I can't do anything," I told the therapist once we got settled, me on a long gray couch across from her half-turned armchair. I wish I could remember her name, but she was young and lovely and listened with gentle patience while I talked for forty-five minutes straight.

"It sounds like you have a mild case of depression," she said near the end of our session. The way she summed it all up made it sound so easy, so fixable. Normal, even.

"Oh, I guess that makes sense," I said. I was on season six of *Buffy*, and our heroine was near-catatonic after rising from the dead. She'd always struggled with her mental health, but in this season it had overtaken her. Maybe Buffy and I really were alike.

"Have you ever tried antidepressants?" the therapist asked, tugging a prescription pad from the crease of her chair.

"No, but I've heard the side effects are no joke." I laughed. I'd read so many books where the main character would go on Zoloft or Prozac and suddenly be unable to have sex or feel much of anything. Was numbness worth the price of admission?

"They can be," she said, scribbling already. "It may take a while to find the right one. I'm really liking Wellbutrin right now. Have you heard of it? It's a norepinephrine-dopamine reuptake inhibitor, so it doesn't cause weight gain or low libido or any of those other common side effects." She handed me the slip of paper, her hand-writing neat and round like a teenage girl's.

I didn't understand what she meant, but I didn't care. I was sold on the idea of a magic pill that would make me functional. "Let's do it."

I walked out of her office and straight to the CVS on Main Street, already happier and more energetic, the mere thought of a solution solving half the problem. For the twenty minutes I waited for the pharmacist to fill the prescription, I walked the aisles, imag-ining the makeup I would wear, the shampoo I would buy. I treated myself to a fresh loofah, a puffy purple cloud, for all the showers I would now take. When the prescription was ready, I took my first pill with a bottle of water right there next to the nail polish.

Outside, the sun was shining, and I smiled at everyone on the sidewalk. Everything would be different now. I'd go for runs in the morning before class, call my friend Lyz from freshman year to go for hikes in the woods off campus, dripping with kudzu. I'd catch up on all my missed assignments. I'd even go to a party or two. Maybe I could *host* a party!

I breezed through the day on a jet stream of possibility. I tidied my room, washed my grubby sheets, took a heaving bag of clothes to the laundry.

That night, I couldn't sleep. My pulse fluttered, faster and faster. For a few panicked minutes, I thought I was having a heart attack, before chalking it up to the frenzy at which I'd worked that day. I tossed and turned all night.

When I woke the next morning, my boisterous energy was gone. I pulled on the same stretchy pants and blue sweater I'd worn the day before, popped another Wellbutrin, and dragged myself to class.

Sitting in Sociology, I blinked my eyes and flared my nostrils every few seconds, as if I'd had too much caffeine. I figured my big day and lack of sleep meant I deserved a rest, so even though my inner voice whispered *lazybones* as I dragged myself back to my apartment, I silenced it with *Buffy* and stayed in bed for the afternoon.

Later, as I tried to fall asleep, I still felt restless and jangly. My new tic that year was rolling my neck and drawing my shoulder blades together. Again and again, I arched into my pillows, pressed the back of my head into the soft down, and rolled it from side to side until a sharp line of pain raced up my skull.

I stopped and sucked air through my nose, filling my lungs and extending my belly like I'd heard on some meditation tape, but my heartbeat sprinted on. After a minute of this I twitched again, flinging my head back like an extra in *Girl, Interrupted*. I was one of those windup chattering teeth, vibrating in erratic circles, going nowhere.

After an hour without relief, I hurled off my blankets and padded to the bathroom for an Advil PM, which blissfully knocked me out.

I STAYED ON WELLBUTRIN for two months, manic and wild during the day, restless at night. The Wellbutrin gave me enough motivation to land a few *B*'s in Sociology, but eventually my frantic, uncontrollable stimming became so unbearable I weaned myself off the medication. Then the nonshowering, nontoothbrushing began again, so I started back on the pills. I flipped and flopped like this until graduation.

I often wonder how I managed well enough in high school but barely made it through college. At fifteen, I woke up at five o'clock every morning to straighten my hair and choose the perfect outfit. I spent an entire seven-hour day bustling among thirty-five hundred other kids, came home and did my homework, and eventually graduated with a strong GPA. Why, when left to my own devices, did I skip half my classes and stop showering?

College is a massive transition for anyone, but especially for autistic teens who have to navigate a hundred transitions at once. We're thrust out of our homes with their comfortable rules and familiarity, suddenly responsible for our every basic need—from doing our laundry to filling prescriptions to feeding ourselves to attending class on time—without the support system that helped us as children.

Steve Silberman, author of *NeuroTribes: The Legacy of Autism and the Future of Neurodiversity*, wrote, "What every parent of a child on the spectrum knows is that, after high school, kids 'age out' of the very meager amount of services that are provided for them. Families often describe this process as 'falling off a cliff.' There are very few programs to help young autistic people transition out of school and into the workplace, even if they're fully capable of working and very eager to work."

Autistic people take longer to complete college and drop out at higher rates—only 41 percent of us graduate, compared to 59 percent of nondisabled students. Like my friend Delia, who attended college twenty years before her autism diagnosis and was forced to drop out after her first semester. "I just felt so exhausted," she texted me when I asked how college had gone for her. "So mentally and physically exhausted that I could barely walk or talk. It was a level of exhaustion I didn't understand. Why was I the only one feeling like that?"

She wasn't the only one, not by a long shot, though I wish women like Delia and me could have been visible to each other— that somebody could have seen what was really happening when I skipped class in favor of another day in bed, when I procrastinated brushing my teeth for the third day in a row, or when I watched Ami's friends dance off to yet another concert or improv show while I surrendered to another night alone.

After learning, at thirty-six, that she is autistic, Delia is back at school, getting her degree in anthropology at Sonoma State. "It's still hard," she told me, "but not in the same way. If I had known I was autistic back then, I would have known how to deal with all this a little better. I grew up thinking I wasn't very smart and was terrified to say that I didn't understand something. Now I know that's not true and I'm not as embarrassed to ask for help. I get extra test time. I'm more confident in asking for what I need."

The transition to college is often a trigger for what's known as *autistic burnout*, a term widely used by members of the autistic community but barely researched by the scientific one. Dr. Dora M. Raymaker was one of the first researchers to look at the topic, defining autistic burnout as a syndrome "resulting from chronic life stress and a mismatch of expectations and abilities without adequate supports." Symptoms are usually long-term, lasting at least three months, and include extreme fatigue, loss of skills, and increased sensory sensitivities.

From the outside, depression and autistic burnout can look identical, so it's no wonder my Davidson therapist was quick to diagnose me with depression and prescribe Wellbutrin, but they are two separate conditions. Burnout is impossible to spot unless you know the patient is autistic.

The main differences are the trigger and the treatment. While depression can be caused by a million things, like stressful life events, genetics, or a chemical imbalance, autistic burnout is almost always due to prolonged masking.

As one participant in the Raymaker study explained, "Long-term camouflaging and masking leaves behind a kind of psychic plaque in the mental and emotional arteries. Like the buildup of physical plaque over time can result in a heart attack or stroke, the buildup of this psychic plaque over time can result in burnout."

In other words, burnout is more likely to happen to autistics who hold themselves to neurotypical standards.

Then there's the treatment. A crucial skill in depression treatment is "behavior activation." It stems from the idea that our behaviors impact our mood—so if our mood is low, changing our behaviors will make us feel better. That's where we start to hear advice like, *Go out and socialize, start a gratitude journal, meditate, take up a sport, take a walk, try yoga, try juicing, call a friend, volunteer. The more you do, the better you'll feel!* I heard that advice from Mom, my therapist, Xander to Buffy, and the self-help books I'd started to read.

The problem is, the activities that benefit depression will often make autistic burnout worse. Behavior activation is the *exact opposite* of what we need to recover. Since autistic burnout is usually worsened by sensory overload, high executive functioning demands, or scheduling changes, the last thing an autistic person needs is more of what got them there. It's like telling someone with a miserable job to spend more time at work.

Which was exactly the roadblock I hit after being diagnosed with depression. The more I tried to claw my way out of it—go to parties! Go to the coffee shop to be around people! Clean my room! Clean my body!—the more depleted I became.

Since starting at Davidson, it felt like someone had handed me three of those lit cartoon bombs and told me to start juggling. If I dropped one, I was dead. After years of keeping them in the air, I wanted to sleep for a century. I had moved beyond exhaustion and into delirium, but everyone around me seemed to be juggling their bombs just fine, so I kept adding more and more to my routine. Here's the yoga bomb! And the frat party bomb! And the coffee shop bomb! And suddenly I was juggling seventeen bombs while everyone told me I should feel better by now.

The best treatment for autistic burnout is sensory detox, unmasking, time with special interests, and rest—gentle, quiet activities we'd never give ourselves permission to do if we didn't know we were autistic.

I attended Davidson thirteen years before my autism diagnosis and three years before the college created its Academic Access and Disability Resources office. Had I known I was autistic, I could have registered for fewer classes each semester, maybe stayed at Davidson an extra year. I could have taken tests in a quiet room instead of submerged in the sounds of pencils scratching at rough paper and the fizzing fluorescent lights overhead. I could have lived alone. I could have embraced sleep instead of punishing myself for needing it. I wouldn't have stepped a single toe inside a frat house.

I recently stumbled across a quote frequently shared in the disability community that stopped me in my tracks. "The problem with trying to fit a square peg into a round hole is not so much the amount of time and effort and frustration of forcing the fit, but that you end up damaging the peg."

And it dawned on me: I might never change, but my environment could.

—9—

Foreign

IN THE WINTER OF MY SOPHOMORE YEAR, FOUR MONTHS BEFORE I turned twenty, I got an email from the dean. Ami and I were in our room, sitting shoulder to shoulder at our respective desks, her clacking away on an essay, while I stared down yet another assignment with so much fatigue that even breathing felt like too much work. Outside our window, the sky was growing dark, but we hadn't yet turned on the lights, so our room was cast in twilight, the glow of our laptops illuminating our faces as if we were about to tell scary stories around a campfire. To make myself feel productive, I refreshed my email for the fifth time in as many minutes. Sitting in my inbox was a message to all sophomores.

"Reminder: Sophomores are required to announce their study abroad decisions by February 1st."

An image of London popped into my head. I'd been a couple of times; once with my family to a flea-infested home exchange in Putney and again in high school for a whirlwind work trip with Mom. I remembered candy apple telephone booths and mossy stone walls and drizzled rain over rolling green lawns. Four years had passed since my summer in Spain, and the memory had taken on a rosy glow. As I'd walked alone through the streets of Santander, I'd transformed into someone free and independent and brave. Abroad, I could be someone other than myself, and so the thought again occurred to me: "Yes. *This* will fix me."

Within the hour I'd found a generic program called IES Abroad, downloaded the application materials, filled them out, and clicked Submit. I didn't even consider another location. I would arrive in London fresh and shiny like a two-pence piece. Everything would be different.

EVERYTHING WAS DIFFERENT. YOU know that saying, "No matter where you go, there you are?" I call bullshit.

In London, I went to every gallery, theater production, tourist attraction, castle, village, forest, and historically significant park bench. I stopped to read every blue plaque on every house and could spot those markers of notable former residents from blocks away. I walked forty-five minutes to my new school instead of taking the tube so I could soak it all in. What was it about this place?

It could have been the people. The women in my program— Rachel, Lauren, and Aly—weren't like the girls I knew in college or Greenwich or Spain. For one thing, they were *mine*, not Ami's or Chelsea's. I was an included, valuable member of the group, not a friend of a friend who awkwardly tagged along.

Aly had a lifelong dream of becoming a librarian, Rachel cared about politics more than anyone I'd ever met, and Lauren was quiet 99 percent of the time, and pure chaos the other 1 percent. She was my adventure buddy, always ready to find the local Hare Krishna monk serving free vegan food outside the University of London. The four of us visited the occasional quiet pub to chat or took a £1 Megabus to various estates around the country. They cared about the things I cared about. When the popular kids got rowdy in the hall kitchen keeping everyone else awake, Rachel was the one to storm in to shut them up before I even had to get out of bed. Halfway across the world, I had found my people.

It could have been the classes. I was reminded that I loved learning when I cared about the material, and I would have been obsessed with every class at my new school regardless of a grade. In one called British Youth Culture, we sat around a long table and nodded thoughtfully while listening to the Cure. British Women Novelists was hosted on the top floor of a creaky old bookstore that smelled like vanilla and damp wood. The History of London was mostly walking tours around a city I traversed by foot anyway.

It could have been London herself. I'd walk through the City of London and look at a thousand-year-old wall and feel like time didn't exist. On free afternoons I took the tube to St. Paul's, where there was this quaint tea shop overlooking the cathedral, just to get a slice of cake and look out the window at the familiar dome that had watched over Londoners for centuries.

Though, let's be honest, it was probably Lewis.

We met on the floor of a hostel in Oslo, Norway. Lauren and I had found a last-minute flight deal for forty pounds, round trip. What was in Oslo? What would we do there for three days? Couldn't tell you then or now, but we were broke and adventurous so we shrugged and booked the tickets.

A few days later, we sat on the grimy hallway floor outside the room we were sharing with twenty other broke and adventurous students, when a couple about our age walked past and must have heard us yell-talking.

"Americans!" said the girl with a strong English accent and gummy smile.

"Ha ha, yeah," I said. Unsure whether this was an insult, I gave a half-hearted *what-can-you-do* shrug.

I glanced at the boy. He was a few years older than me, and he smiled with his mouth open, showing a cute gap between his front teeth. His eyes were the blue a child would use in a coloring-book image of a prince, startling even behind his narrow glasses. His face was rough with a day or two of dark scruff that I suspected was permanent, and he wore, on this frigid Norwegian night, a slim brown coat and a messenger bag slung across his chest.

"Hi," he said. I couldn't place his accent.

They joined us on the floor, our four backs pressed against the concrete wall, and within minutes I had fallen in love with this shy boy. Turned out he was a Kiwi, and I kept asking him to say words so I could compare our pronunciation. At twenty, I knew nothing about New Zealand, so I flung questions at him like grenades.

"Is it sunny year-round?"

"No, we have four seasons, sometimes all in one day, but it's lovely in the summer."

"You look pretty tan actually," I said, eyeing him up and down like a little pervert.

"My hands may be tan but the *rist* of me is white." He pulled the sleeve of his coat up an inch to show me the pale skin on his forearm.

"Your wrist?"

"The riiiist," he said slower, gesturing broadly to himself.

"Oh, the *rest*!" I laughed. Then blushed furiously as I imagined *the rest* of him. Oh boy, was I in trouble.

Something about his quiet yet polite demeanor made me turn up the dial of my own deeply hidden charm. I wanted to show off who I had become here: cute, fun, and up for anything. With barely a day's notice I'd flown to a country I knew nothing about—look at how interesting and spontaneous I am!

For hours we sat talking about nothing and everything. His companion, Jane, wasn't his girlfriend but a friendly coworker, and she and Lauren sat rolling their eyes at each other while I threw myself at Lewis like a fly against a window. I learned that not only did Lewis and Jane also live in London, but their office was on the same block as my internship at the Royal Academy of Arts.

"Sweet as!" Lewis said when I told him.

"Sweet . . . ass?" I asked. Was he making a pass at me? *Ohthankgod.*

"No!" He turned red. "Sweet AS. As in . . . as."

"What the hell does *that* mean?"

"Oh—um. Everything! *Thank you. You're welcome. No worries. That's great.* It's kind of a catchall."

"Well then, sweet ass!" I said, laughing. We exchanged info and promised to meet up once we returned to England.

"I'm obsessed with him," I said to Lauren, after they'd left.

She laughed. "I can see that."

"He's so easy to talk to. And *cute.*" I sighed dramatically. "I must seduce him."

"Well, ask him out when we get home."

"I will!"

When Lauren and I arrived back in London, I hopped straight on Facebook to search for Lewis. There he was, smiling into the sun, a snow-covered mountain in the background. He was even cuter than I remembered. I added him as a friend and sent a super subtle, not-at-all obvious message . . .

1. i am happy to report that you are the only lewis john-sullivan in existence (actually, on facebook, but whatever—same thing)
2. your picture makes me want to be your best friend
3. lauren and i have been saying a) "sweet as" at every possible opportunity, and b) your name over and over again trying to get her to say it right.
4. i like lists.

Oh my god, flirting in your twenties. What a time to be alive.

At least it worked, because suddenly we were meeting up weekly during our lunch breaks to walk around Green Park, messaging each other links to Flight of the Conchords videos, and standing slightly too close on tube rides to various trendy pubs while I wondered what it would be like to kiss him. After a month of friendly-but-flirty hangouts, I still had no idea if he was interested in me. The more ambivalent he acted, the more I pushed, performing the role of an over-the-top, sexually liberated American.

One night, sick of waiting for him to make a move, I invited him for dinner at my tiny shared-dorm kitchen. I cooked a quinoa stir-fry; he brought a bottle of New Zealand wine. I talked at him for the entire date until, both of us full and awkward and a little nervous, he kissed me at last, probably to shut me up. It was mostly chaste, but my body turned into a shaken bottle of seltzer, and I wrapped my arms around his neck to pull him closer. I asked why he took so long, and he paused before admitting he had limited experience in these things and had no idea what to do.

"Most of my friends are girls," he said. "They're not really lining up around the block to date me."

Their loss, I thought.

My journals from that month are filled with page after page about this nerdy Kiwi boy: "He's such a good listener. He asks questions, then he sits and stares at me when I talk and then he'll remember what I said weeks later by referencing it again." (My bar for men was sky high.)

On our first sleepover we stayed awake until three o'clock in the morning, talking about feminism and vegetarianism and every other ism, until our eyes grew heavy and we fell asleep, arms and legs sprawled over and under each other on my twin bed.

"What is happening to me?" I wrote after he left the next morning. "I really *really* like this guy."

As I dotted that last period my phone dinged with a text from him. "Last night was . . . quite wow." I clutched the phone to my heart.

I extended that first semester in London to two. I'd even started showering again—it was easy when I had the crackling excitement of new love to keep me clean. Why would I go back to Davidson when I had all this?

By that January, Rachel, Aly, and Lauren had returned to their real lives and were replaced by another group of young and eager Americans. I had a life in London away from the program, so I didn't try to befriend them. I don't even remember my second roommate's name; that's how often I was there. But it didn't matter, because I had Lewis and his ragtag gang of locals and expats, and I had this city, which delighted me at every corner.

After class, I'd take the tube to Aldgate East while listening to playlists Lewis had made, introducing me to bands that made me feel cool just to know their names. I climbed the stairs out of the station and into the dark streets of London, Anohni and the Johnsons crooning in my ears while I walked the ten minutes to Lewis's apartment, which sat atop a curry house. He slept on an air mattress in the living room, too cheap to pay for a room to himself. His roommates gave us privacy when they could, leaving the space dark and quiet except for the yellow streetlights pouring a puddle of warm light over the hardwood and the sluice of cars through the rain on the streets below.

From the moment we met, an expiration date was built into our relationship. Even with my semester extension, I'd eventually have to return home to finish college. Our bubble was fragile, and we both knew it would pop, but for now, it was delicate and bright and shiny and neither of us dared exhale.

By April, I was dizzy and breathless. No way could I leave *now*! I couldn't afford to stay in my study abroad program, so I applied for a six-month working visa for under-thirties, got a job at a Tex-Mex restaurant in Trafalgar Square (yes, it was as offensive as you might imagine), and moved into a council flat near Mile End with a random South African guy I met on Gumtree, the UK version of Craigslist. I stayed for Lewis, and for the me I was with him. Living in London made me wonder whether my problem was that I didn't belong in America. Maybe I was born in the wrong country, or maybe my personality was better suited to being a strange person in a strange land.

Years later, I spoke with Sarah Hendrickx, an autistic author and speaker, about this contradiction. How could a small American college experience have destabilized me so completely, while moving to a major global city unlocked a version of me who was resourceful and energetic? Sarah lives in France, though she's originally from England. Over the phone she told me, "I know many autistic people who feel more comfortable outside their own culture. You still have to look for the social cues, but you're not actually expected to get them all right. I'm not autistic in France; I'm just foreign. It's a massive liberation."

Several other autistics have written about this phenomenon, including Devon Price in *Unmasking Autism* when he wrote, "No one sees you as an 'overly sensitive' disabled person if you're constantly traveling the world."

In London I could be eccentric and brassy, but that didn't mean I was inherently broken—I was just American. After years of feeling inadequate, navigating London on my own made me feel confident and grown-up, even *special.* The history of the city and constant barrage of newness kept my brain engaged and away from self-hatred. And to be loved by this boy, in his quiet way, meant things must be finally clicking into place.

ON MY TWENTY-FIRST BIRTHDAY, Lewis and I took a weekend getaway to the gray coastal town of Bournemouth. Even though I was of legal drinking age in the United Kingdom, and we could have gone out to a bar, we bought a bottle of Malibu rum and a chocolate cake from Tesco that we picked at with plastic forks while sitting on the curb of a small park. We walked along the blustery beach, holding hands and bracing ourselves against the wind until we were too cold to stay outside.

Back in our hotel room, Lewis sat me on the floral bedspread and handed me a small box.

"For me?" I asked.

"Of course. Just something from home."

Inside was a greenstone pendant shaped like a pear with a twist at the top. Lewis had told me how special pounamu was to New Zealanders and Māori culture. You can't buy it for yourself; it must be gifted. Tucked underneath the pendant was a printed slip of paper. "The twist represents the joining of two people for eternity. They sometimes move away from each other on their own journeys, but they will always come together again sharing their lives and blending to become one."

Davidson was 3,976 miles away, and my frayed connection to that place snapped, releasing its hold. Here was a life that was mine.

EVENTUALLY IT WAS AUGUST again. I'd been in England for a year, but I'd burned through every extension and visa to do it. I had to go back to finish my last two semesters at Davidson.

On the day of my flight home, Lewis rode the train with me to the airport, my giant suitcase bulging between my legs, our knees pressed together, hands clasped so tight I couldn't feel my fingers. I watched my beloved city fly past outside the train windows. Every patch of gray sky, every tenement and motorway, was the most gloriously beautiful thing I'd ever seen.

The closer we inched to Heathrow, the more my chest threatened to collapse in on itself. I gazed at Lewis next to me, and his eyes were unfocused and red around the rims. He caught me staring and pressed his lips together before squeezing my hand.

At the airport, we walked, slow and wordless, to the security line. When he couldn't take me any farther, we turned to each other. I flung my arms around him and sobbed.

"I can't do this. I can't go back."

"You can," he muttered into my ear. "I love you."

We kissed then, furious and damp, vowing to stay together. He waited as I made my way through security, and I looked back at him one last time before turning the corner and leaving him behind. One of us would find our way to the other; we just needed to get through the next year.

—10—

Buzzkill

LEWIS VISITED ME TWICE AT DAVIDSON, BUT THE MAGIC WAS MUTED, as if muffled by a weighted blanket. Maybe we worked only in the drizzly, romantic streets of London and couldn't survive the wider world or the reality of my true nature. As much as I loved him, he didn't know the real me—the girl who didn't leave the house for days or brush her teeth or go to class or do her homework. He didn't know who I'd been before he saw me laughing on the hostel floor.

We broke up in January, were back together by Valentine's, and called it off again in June. I graduated and briefly moved to New York, until Manhattan's constant haze of urine and the dissonant yell of saxophones on every corner sent me running back to Lewis and London one last, heartbreaking time.

By then Lewis had moved to Leytonstone, a gray, villagey neighborhood nearly an hour outside Central London full of chicken shops and off-licenses and one pub, where he could afford his own room in a narrow brick flat squashed between a dozen other narrow brick flats. Since I'd moved across the world to be with him, I didn't even bother looking for my own place: I hung my dresses next to his work shirts and called it mine.

The Leytonstone house was a revolving door of cousins and

friends who were either related to Lewis, had gone to college with Lewis, or were dating someone related to or college friends with Lewis. They invited me to every costume party, pub trivia, camping trip, indie concert, barbecue, and poker night, laughing and drinking with casual intimacy as I watched, wishing I were anywhere else. I hadn't noticed this before we lived together, or maybe it hadn't existed in the early days of our love cocoon where we didn't need or want anyone except each other, but now that we shared a home, I was realizing Lewis had a never-ending desire to socialize. I would have been perfectly happy spending evenings alone with him watching movies or making veggie curries.

I usually stayed at the flat and stewed in resentment that he needed more than me. Some nights, in an attempt to silence the girl who had moped around Davidson like a lazy ghost, I forced myself to tag along, which went about as well as you can imagine.

One night, Lewis invited me out to meet an old friend of his from New Zealand. My British visa was only temporary, so we'd decided to move to his hometown of Auckland, where I could live and work freely. It was a big move, so he thought it'd be nice for me to make some friends before we arrived. I was in the middle of trying to make it as a freelance writer, which usually meant twelve-hour days for terrible pay, so I was sluggish and uninterested in leaving the flat, never mind spending an hour on the tube, then needing to focus all my energy and attention on conversations with people I didn't care about, but I pushed through, because that's what people in their twenties do.

We met at a small British pub, but it felt like a Taylor Swift concert. Lewis and his friends were seated at a tall round table near the center of the room, and they gave big smiles when they spotted me. The music thumped through my body like a hammer and I couldn't manage a smile back. *Cool start, Marian.* I made an excuse to grab a drink and tried to pull myself together.

My personal version of hell is trying to get a bartender's attention.

Was everyone else given a manual on how to do this? Do you push between two people chatting on barstools? Do you shout? Lift a hand? (Is that rude?) And where's the line? Is it like a four-way stop sign, and if so, are we supposed to let the person to our right go before us, or the person who arrived first? But at a long bar full of twenty people sitting and ten others waiting, *how do you keep track*? *WHAT ARE THE RULES?*

By the time I got my half-pint of cider, I was clamoring to go home. It felt so unsettling and quivery, all that activity, and I was frantic to be rid of it, like someone had just announced there was a spider in my hair.

I scrambled onto the tall stool between Lewis's cousin Charlie and his Kiwi friend Isa. She acknowledged me with a small half nod. Isa had a septum piercing and an undercut that screamed *I am anarchy! I am chaos! I make sweeping contrarian statements just to start an argument!* I teetered on the stool next to her like a child.

Isa and Lewis were deep in conversation about obscure music, so I gripped my sweating glass of cider and let the cold seep into my bones and the condensation trickle onto the cardboard coaster below.

Charlie sat to my left. I loved Charlie, but he was goofy in a way I didn't understand. Next to him I felt obtuse and humorless, but behind the resting bitch face my brain was just trying to decipher the joke.

Lewis's friends usually talked about things I didn't care about, and without a way to meaningfully contribute I often sat silently, looking uptight and dour while I scanned my mental files to pull up a conversation—any conversation—I'd heard in my twenty-three years to parrot back to them. If I couldn't find one, I'd spiral on how to participate. Should I start a separate conversation? How exactly does one do that? Was I supposed to ask follow-up questions? How, if I didn't know or care about the topic? Should I wait until they asked *me* a question? Was that selfish? Oh, but now there was this awkward silence—could they feel it too? The longer it went on, the worse it got, the more pressure I felt to say the right thing . . .

"Do you—?"

"How long—?"

Charlie and I spoke at the same time, and oh god that was even *worse*.

Lewis squeezed my knee under the table. I rested my head on his shoulder and wondered whether he could tell I was floundering. His gentle awareness of me in any room sometimes made it feel like I had to perform for him too. I knew how much he wanted me to get along with his friends, but every time we went out together, I let him down.

"You all right?" he whispered.

"Yup," I said, trying to keep it casual, but it came out snippy. My bones ached. I couldn't produce a single ounce of energy or enthusiasm. *Okay, that's okay, it's one hour*, I told myself. *You can do this. Sit quietly and listen; you don't need to say anything.*

"How's work?" asked Isa, looking at Lewis.

"Yeah, you know. Work." He laughed and waved off the question before taking a gulp of his beer. "How's the family?"

The seconds dragged behind me like taffy, and I disappeared into the red-and-beige flocked wallpaper. I reached my focus out to their conversation, but there were too many happening at the surrounding tables and the speeding Rolodex of my brain kept flipping through them without capturing their meaning.

"Have you heard the new Nick Cave?"

"No, I'm not heading home for the holiday."

"Yeah, it's brilliant."

"Oi! Mate, you forgot your wallet!"

"Ah, that's a shame."

My body took over. I pushed up from the table, almost tipping our beers, and whispered to Lewis, "I'm sorry, I have to go." I fled without saying goodbye to Charlie or Isa.

Once I was anonymous on the streets of London, I allowed myself to dissolve, tears streaking down my face and landing on the pavement. *Why can everyone else so easily keep up a conversation? Do they actually like this? How can they have so much fun at a bar while it feels like torture to me? And why can't I muscle through?* Lewis was going to leave me, I knew it.

With that thought, a hand brushed my lower back and I turned to see him, his blue eyes searching, his eyebrows furrowed. Before he had a chance to speak, I sputtered, "It's fine, I'm fine. Go back inside."

"I can't go back inside when you're out here like this."

"I don't—I don't want to ruin your night. Go be with your friends."

"Marian, stop." His tone teetered on the edge of anger, the flash of a knife. "What do you need? Do you want to go home?"

"I'm overwhelmed. It's too loud." I buried my face in his chest, and he wrapped his arms around me. "I'm so sorry," I sobbed. "I'm so sorry. I keep ruining your social life."

"You're not ruining my social life." Behind his comforting words and his warm body, I sensed his disappointment. He hadn't seen Isa in years, and he'd managed to hang out with her for thirty minutes before his touchy American girlfriend ran out of the bar in tears. I imagined Charlie and Isa giving each other pointed stares. *She's a little dramatic, isn't she?* they'd whisper. *Poor Lewis.*

The worst part of it all wasn't even the overwhelm. The worst part was that I knew exactly what was expected of me on a theoretical level, but I couldn't force my body into doing the movements. Like when your foot goes numb and you know you need to stand and shake it out, but your body won't cooperate.

I wanted to make Lewis happy, but more than anything, I wanted to be the person I'd been during our first year together. Outside this British pub, I couldn't sense her anywhere. Maybe London Marian wasn't real. Maybe she was a role I'd played on a temporary adventure to the other side of the world, another mask I'd been wearing.

From the preening newness of our early relationship to the yearning agony of long distance, Lewis and I had been together two years before he met the woman who skulked underneath it all. By that time, it was too late. We'd already booked tickets for a new life together in New Zealand.

WE ARRIVED IN AUCKLAND that December, to a sky so broad and blue I felt like we'd landed inside a kitschy tropical snow globe. It was nearly summer in the southern hemisphere and the breeze was warm and grassy. The looming red ball of the sun seemed bigger, lower, more present than I'd ever seen it back home.

We'd be living with Lewis's parents, Greg and Sharon, in the lush suburb of Browns Bay. "Have just bought you guys a bed today!!" Sharon wrote me in an email the week before our flight. "Looking forward to your arrival, Flower!!" She called me pet names like Petal and Love and Flower. When we met in person, she put her hands on either side of my face and sighed to Lewis, "Look how lovely she is!"

Living with your boyfriend's parents is the setup for a sitcom or a nightmare, but Greg and Sharon were the friendliest, most accommodating roommates on earth. It was me who was the problem.

I hated New Zealand immediately. The internet was too slow. Groceries were too expensive. It was hot, but no one had air-conditioning. The coastal trail up Rangitoto was paved with volcanic rock and I couldn't get my footing. The house was full of cockroaches.

I've always been terrified of bugs, especially cockroaches. At Abuelo's house in Puerto Rico, they were big enough to saddle up and ride. Their thin legs and long, hard bodies sent me into immediate hysterics. In Browns Bay, they were everywhere.

On our first morning I walked downstairs to see one flailing on its back inside the cool metal bowl of an old-fashioned kitchen scale. A sprinkling of flour had been left behind in the bottom of the bowl, and as it wriggled, its legs became coated in fine white powder. The red arm of the scale barely registered its weight. The shriek that came out of me was obscene.

Sharon came running and I pointed toward the counter. She

grabbed a paper towel, then plucked the bug out of the bowl and tossed it into the trash. The ease with which she handled it made me feel like I was being hysterical.

The next day I pulled open the living room curtains, and a cockroach darted from between the folds. The day after that, another greeted me at the front door like some monstrous Kafkaesque butler.

Every morning I peeked out of our bedroom and examined the ceiling, the walls, the corners of the floors, before moving through the house like a one-woman SWAT team. At night, convinced I heard scuttling, I turned on all the lights and shook Lewis awake, forcing him to scan every surface for roaches. We never found one that way, of course. My SWAT routine didn't eliminate the worst parts of my fear—the anticipation and unpredictability. Roaches darted out and surprised me only in the moments I let my guard down, skittering over my feet as we sat outside on the twilit patio or lying in wait on shower walls. Each time I leaped back as if I'd gripped a live wire. As the weeks passed, I started waking up braced for electrocution.

My panic and unhappiness impacted everyone in the house. Lewis and I were chatting on our bed one night, my back against the headboard, him perched on the edge of the mattress with his hand on my knee, when his eyes darted to the wall behind me. He froze, and said slowly, "Don't look behind you."

My stomach lurched and I tried to breathe through the terror.

"Walk out of the room, I'll take care of it," he said. I nodded and ran out the door, shame trailing behind me as I fled.

On Christmas Eve, Lewis's entire family was visiting—his brother and sister-in-law, her parents, a smattering of family friends. After dinner, I left to use the bathroom, and when I returned, they were all whispering, their heads leaning together over the table. Lewis's brother glanced toward me, and silence fell across the room.

"What's going on?" I asked.

"It's nothing, don't worry about it," said Lewis. He bit the corner of his lip and looked toward his mother.

"I'm going to worry about it," I said. "I feel super self-conscious."

"It's about the cockroaches, Petal," said Sharon gently.

"Ah," I sighed out. I didn't want to hear anymore, not about the roaches and definitely not about how unreasonably I was behaving. I already knew. I had arrived from America and inflicted a virus upon this kind, unsuspecting family.

When we weren't home, Lewis was determined to make me fall in love with New Zealand. He dragged me to black sand beaches, hidden rainforests, and volcanic islands, but I lagged behind, tripping over rocks and muttering to myself, *This is horrible, this is awful, why does anyone like this country?* I looked out on sweeping vistas and saw nothing. It might as well have been in black-and-white.

My disgust was obvious to anyone who spent more than five minutes in my delightful presence. I've never been able to keep my opinions to myself. The second I have a thought, it forms a rock in my mouth and I can't speak or swallow until I spit it out. Sometimes this works to my advantage by making people laugh or helping them feel like they can trust me because they always know what I'm thinking; more often, it takes them aback. I bulldoze over their opinions and hurt their feelings. (Classic Autism Symptom #457: People think you're being rude or critical when you don't mean to be.)

By month three, all semblance of my filter had disappeared. I criticized everything with great enthusiasm. One night, Greg and Sharon pulled together a beautiful dinner, which the four of us were enjoying outside. Something got us started on the state of women's rights. I'd recently graduated with a minor in gender studies, so I had a lot of passionate opinions. Greg asked an innocent question I can't remember, but at that point in my life I took it to mean that the white man was about to mansplain feminism and I leaped down his throat, got so flustered I couldn't talk, and stormed inside, my dinner half-finished on my plate.

A month or so later, Greg and Sharon adopted a miniature

schnauzer named Daisy. Small dogs are not my favorite, and I missed the drooling rambunctious springer spaniel from my childhood, whose tongue lolled to the side and whose butt wiggled whenever she saw us. Daisy was new to the family and a little reserved, but instead of keeping my dislike of her to myself, I called her "soulless" to Sharon's face and wrote an eight-hundred-word essay on my blog about how much I hated her.

Sharon pulled me into the dining room that night and gently explained, "That article you wrote really hurt my feelings, Petal."

I apologized, but I'm sure it came out forced and resigned. I took the blog post down, but the damage had already been done.

Despite it all, Greg and Sharon kept trying to connect with me. I got a part-time job at a local bakery, and after hours on my feet mixing batter and making mediocre flat whites, I had barely enough energy to shower the icing out of my hair, never mind chat with my pseudo in-laws. When I came home in the afternoons, I was almost always met with questions: *How are you, Flower? Do you want to go for a walk? Can I make you a snack?* I'd grunt out an excuse and sprint upstairs.

Later, my stomach churned with hunger, but what if I ran into Sharon in the kitchen and she wanted to have a heart-to-heart? I'd lie in bed, listening for the slam of the front door and the rattle of her car pulling out of the driveway. If she didn't leave, I resigned my-self to going hungry because I was so terrified of the conversation. I felt uncomfortable anywhere except my room, but even that I shared with Lewis, and I'd stopped feeling comfortable around him too.

Lewis couldn't understand my bewildering behavior. We stopped talking, stopped touching, and the air around us became heavy and toxic, laden with the things left unsaid. It would only be a matter of time before one of us spoke aloud the truth—this wasn't working—but it sure as hell wouldn't be me, eight thousand miles from home. I clung to Lewis like a life raft. The girl he met on the

Norwegian hostel floor was dead and buried under a mountain of blankets and a boxed set of *Alias*.

WHEN I TELL OTHER disabled people about this period in my life, one word comes up more than any other: *spoons*.

"It sounds like you didn't have the spoons to socialize," and "If you used up all your spoons at work, it makes sense that you wouldn't have any left to deal with a cockroach showing up."

Spoon Theory was created by Christine Miserandino, a writer and advocate living with lupus. She came up with the metaphor while at a diner with a friend. Her friend asked what it was like living with a chronic illness, and on a whim, Christine grabbed all the spoons from their table and another, and handed them to her friend. "Most people wake up with an endless supply of spoons," she explained, "but here, for this experiment, you have twelve." She asked her friend to walk her through her day, and for each activity Christine took away a spoon. Getting up and brushing your teeth costs a spoon. Showering costs a spoon—two spoons if you blow-dry your hair and put on makeup. Making breakfast costs two spoons because you have to decide what to cook and then spend time cooking it. "When your 'spoons' are gone, they are gone," Christine said.

Since Christine's infamous blog post, *spoons* has become a shorthand for the experience of living with limited physical, emotional, and psychosocial resources. If you're disabled, every choice must be deliberate. If you're running low on spoons and haven't eaten dinner, you need to do some speedy math to determine whether you have the spoons to cook but not clean up, have the resources to ask for help, or should skip dinner entirely—risking your spoon count for the next day.

This math is possible only if we know we're disabled. Many of us live decades blowing through our spoons by lunchtime and wondering why we're always so depleted.

In 2011, cockroaches stole all my spoons. Living with a chatty couple in their sixties put me in the negative. I had nothing left for Lewis or politeness or making friends or exploring this beautiful country I wanted to call home.

Lewis and I stayed this way for six excruciating months. "We need to get out of here," I told him. "Living in this house is ruining us." One by one, our London roommates had also moved back to New Zealand, so the five of us rented a sky-blue cottage a few blocks from the Auckland Zoo. In the early mornings, I heard lions roaring through our bedroom window.

Established in our own space, Lewis and I settled more deeply into a life. I left the bakery and got a full-time job at a marketing agency staffed entirely by twentysomethings, and Lewis decided to go back to school to become a software engineer. Our new house didn't have a single cockroach.

And yet things between us didn't improve. I still came home after work and snuck past our roommates so they wouldn't rope me into a last-minute concert or "family dinner." Lewis would walk into our bedroom to find me under the covers, but I didn't want connection; I wanted solitude. We were living together, but our lives had split in two, and without the threat of cockroaches or his parents, I no longer had an excuse for my behavior. When I looked at him, I only saw the ways I hadn't lived up to the best, most interesting version of myself.

Two months later, he sat me down on our rumpled bed.

"We don't act like two people who love each other," he told me.

My stomach lurched. I had known this was coming, but it was more romantic to pretend that love was all we needed. It didn't matter that I was equally miserable; I couldn't stand the thought of losing him.

"I know," I admitted. "But I *love* you. This is a blip! Everyone says relationships are hard. We've had so much transition this year— living with your parents, my lack of friends, my new job, our new house, your program. We probably need to settle in a bit longer. I know it must be so hard living with me, I've been such a pill. Maybe I just need my own friends. I can start going out with my coworkers, join a choir or something. We were so good in London. I think I need to figure out who I am *here*."

He hesitated before sighing out, "I love you too, but—"

"Then why aren't you trying harder to save us?" I snapped.

"I don't think it's supposed to be *this* hard," he said.

Our breakup was long and painful, the kind where you fumble in the dark, bumping into each other as you try to find the exit. For a week Lewis slept on our old air mattress while I lay alone in the empty space of our bedroom. He snuck in one night to grab an extra pillow, and as he passed, I reached for his hand and begged him to stay.

For a moment I thought he'd climb in next to me. "I don't think that's a good idea," he whispered, before disappearing back out the door.

I had nowhere to go, no reason to return back to the States, no friends to crash with in New Zealand, and so I turned to adventure—the only place I had ever really liked myself.

I had just enough money to buy a one-way ticket to Australia, where I would stay with strangers for free using a new website called Couchsurfing. If I couldn't find a host, I'd volunteer on farms in exchange for a place to stay. I told Lewis I'd be back in two months. If I could resurrect London Marian, maybe he would love me again.

I flew to Melbourne and crashed with a thirtysomething named Amanda, who gifted me with two days alone in her apartment. As a thank-you, I did her laundry, but I immediately overflowed her washing machine and spent most of those two days walking back and forth to the laundromat, arms heavy with sopping towels. I volunteered on a bush cleanup crew in the Dandenong Ranges and rode in a bumpy van full of strangers. We watched open-mouthed as kangaroos bounded in the distance and the sun rose golden over the hills. I hitched a ride to Sydney with a girl named Carmen who'd gotten a new job and was moving in with her sister. We stopped in

Canberra for ice lollies. In Sydney I spent a week in the decked-out spare room of a guy named Daniel who bought me a box of pastries one morning "just because."

During month two I flew to Queenstown, New Zealand, where I was picked up in an unmarked van by an American guy named Rick who made big money doing special effects for *The Lord of the Rings*. He'd used said money to buy acres of land to rebuild native forests. I spent a month there in Paradise (literally, that's the name of the town), planting trees on a hillside and sleeping in a six-by-six-foot cabin with a giant picture window that overlooked a snow-covered mountain range called the Remarkables (yes, also the real name—it turns out New Zealand is breathtaking?).

Alone and free from the pressure of performing the woman Lewis expected me to be, I found her again. Turns out, I was brave only when there was no other option. I was charming only when there was no one left to impress. I could see beauty in the world only when there was no one watching for my reaction.

But I missed Lewis. I missed the stability of belonging to someone. This trip had only solidified my conviction that we were perfect together and everything would be better once I'd found myself. I'd read *Eat Pray Love*, I knew how this was supposed to work.

Without internet in Paradise I spent every night writing a speech designed to convince Lewis to give us another shot. We hadn't spoken or texted while I was away, but every night I wrote and practiced all seventeen melodramatic paragraphs about how you have to destroy something to rebuild it stronger, and that love like this only comes around once in a lifetime. I reflected on every wonderful memory we'd made together and memorized the entire thing. I knew that if I said the right words, in the right way, everything would be okay.

I flew back to Auckland in early October. After weeks lugging a fertilizer backpack up the steep hills of the South Island, I was windswept and muscular. I spent my last forty dollars on a salon blowout and wore my favorite flowy summer dress and a calf-length crocheted cardigan that made me feel like I belonged on the pages of *Boho Living*. I was the picture of casual, chill adventurer. *Remember me, Lewis? I'm the girl you flirted with on the hostel floor.*

We met on a bench in Albert Park next to a Victorian cast-iron fountain. It was windy and too cold for my outfit. My teeth clattered as I started my speech.

Lewis didn't interrupt, just watched me with his intense blue eyes as I filibustered our relationship. I looked at the messenger bag slung across his chest, the same one he'd had since Oslo.

When I was done, his expression conveyed kindness, but not passion or love. His tone was gentle and sad.

"I'm *so* happy for you," he said. Then he paused, as if looking for the right words, though he didn't need a month of practice to express himself. "But we've both earned ourselves some amazing opportunities outside of each other that deserve our full focus. I'll always look back on our time together with a lot of joy, even if it's painful now. You've enriched my life, helped me grow, and parts of me feel so intertwined with you it's scary. For now though, that's where I need to leave things."

I nodded, and kept nodding. I looked across the park toward Sky Tower, piercing the gray clouds above it. The wind sprayed a mist from the fountain into my hair. I wrapped my arms around myself. The birds and the breeze and the bubbling water whittled into a tiny pinprick of focus, and I couldn't see any of it, only the future with him zipping past me and into the ether.

"Okay," I said, still nodding over and over. It was all I could manage.

I wanted to hate him for giving up on us. I wanted to keep fighting until he caved. But I didn't hate him because I didn't blame him. I wouldn't love me either.

—11—

Highly Sensitive Person

THE CLINIC WAS A TEN-MINUTE WALK FROM MY NEW OFFICE IN SAN Francisco, through a highway underpass crammed with tents, around the corner from a Whole Foods. The waiting room looked like a West Elm catalog, with soft gray couches, midcentury coffee tables, and abstract art in muted earth tones. It was empty when I arrived, so I sat on a couch to wait. A white noise machine hummed in the corner, and I felt a space open in my chest.

After five minutes, I heard a door creak open somewhere down the hallway, then footsteps coming toward me. Then Laura appeared. My new therapist towered over me, her long, blown-out red hair swishing around her elbows like a nineties commercial for Herbal Essences.

"You must be Marian," she said, with a relaxed smile. "Follow me."

I trailed behind her into a cozy office. Eyelet curtains drifted in the breeze. I took a seat on the couch across from what was clearly the Therapist's Chair; a yellow legal pad perched on the arm, and a steaming mug of tea was positioned on the side table, like an Instagram vignette of self-care.

I sat on my hands and leaned forward, waiting for her to begin. Laura cupped her mug. My eyes darted to the art above her—a photograph of unnaturally blue waves crashing onto a pink sand beach. I knew I was supposed to look in her eyes, so I flicked between her and the photo. I stared at her for a few seconds—*hold two three four five*—then looked away.

"Why don't you tell me why you're here," Laura said, interrupting my counting. She took a sip of her tea.

"Oh god, how much time do you have? Oh right, fifty-five minutes. *Ha ha ha ha ha.*" I laughed too loud.

She rewarded me with a smile but stayed silent.

"If I could sum it up," I said, collecting myself, "I'd say that I feel frustrated and angry all the time, but my life is going great. I don't know why I'm so miserable."

"What do you mean by miserable?"

"Well, take my work. I just moved here after living in New Zealand for two years. I got offered this extremely cool job at a travel company, which is basically just a clubhouse for adults. There's a swing hanging from the rafters and one of those nylon parachutes they use at preschools pinned to the ceiling. They feed us breakfast, lunch, and dinner, all catered by this actual professional chef and we eat together 'as a family' and stay at the office all day, but that's never really been my thing."

"What's not your thing?"

"Socializing? Working twelve hours a day? I feel like I'm supposed to be over-the-moon thrilled with this setup. I mean, they relocated me here from across the world, and this was supposed to be the start of my real life with a real career, but I'm so . . . exhausted."

I was surprised to feel pinpricks behind my eyes. I hadn't realized how tired I was. Well, enough to know I should see a therapist for the first time since college, but I've never been a person who cries around people, never mind someone I met five minutes ago. Yet here I was about to dissolve on the couch of this redheaded goddess with long, beaded earrings.

I waited for her to tell me I was being childish. That I had it good and if I would stop focusing on the negative for two seconds, happiness would follow.

Laura was the third therapist I'd seen that month.

Number one was Shanti, who'd come highly recommended by a colleague. "She does mindfulness-based somatic therapy. You'll love her."

About ten minutes into my first session with Shanti, in an office full of mismatched Urban Outfitters tapestries and incense, she interrupted my monologue. "Look at the crystals in front of you. Which one calls to you?"

"Calls to me?"

"Speaks to how you're feeling right now."

"Um . . ." My eyes scanned the brimming table between us—an amethyst that looked like rock candy, a dark-gray metallic hematite, a small wooden bowl filled with tigereye. Pretty, but did they represent my *emotions*? I squinted at the crystals, trying to feel something.

"Don't think too hard," she said. "Feel."

I couldn't stand her attention, so I grabbed the prettiest crystal: a rough hunk the color of pink lemonade.

"Rose quartz, lovely choice." She placed her right palm over her chest. "Rose quartz is connected to your heart chakra. It can help you release negative emotions. Close your eyes."

I did as I was told. My hand was damp and I wanted to wipe it on my pants. I worried that if I put the quartz back all sweaty, Shanti would pick it up and gag—

"Focus on the negative feelings you came in with today," she said. "Focus on how you *want* to feel."

I didn't know how I wanted to feel, I just knew which feelings I wanted to disappear: discontent, exhaustion, irritation, loneliness, overwhelm. That felt like an unreasonable request to make of a rock.

I left Shanti's office still discontented and exhausted and irritated and lonely and overwhelmed, but with a new layer of guilt because I'd done therapy wrong.

Therapist number two was at the top of a list on my insurance website. Dr. Cynthia was a harsh-looking woman in her sixties who practiced out of an enormous wood-paneled office across town. She reminded me of my mother's mother, a large, formidable woman who always sounded exasperated.

At the end of our session, Dr. Cynthia told me I was "enormously privileged" and I should count my blessings every night. A gratitude journal would cure me.

By twenty-five I'd lived in Spain, England, New Zealand, and Australia. After my breakup with Lewis, I'd stayed in New Zealand another year. I'd hiked the Tongariro Crossing and made friends with couchsurfers; I'd graduated from a six-month yoga teacher training and ridden on the back of some guy's motorcycle through the serpentine roads of the Coromandel. Before I left, I managed to secure my dream job at Couchsurfing headquarters in San Francisco *and* a palatial two-bedroom sublet in the bougie neighborhood of Noe Valley. Mom visited that spring and gaped at my apartment. "I hope you know how lucky you are," she said.

I *was* lucky, I did know, which is why my unhappiness terrified me. If I couldn't be happy now, with all this, what was even the point in trying?

So I didn't go back to Dr. Cynthia either.

I found Laura through a cooperative clinic. After a forty-five-minute interview with their intake coordinator, I heard: "Laura will be *perfect* for you." She took my insurance info and scheduled me for the following week.

Sitting across from Laura, I lurched into an explanation of why I was there while part of me braced for judgment.

"It doesn't matter how hard I try," I said, "no matter where I go or live, I end up in the exact same place. Friendless, overwhelmed, exhausted, twitchy. I get home every night and collapse into bed and watch too much TV. Sometimes I can't even get up to shower, and just living a normal life feels like it's so much more *work* than for most people."

"What makes you think most people aren't overwhelmed?"

"I don't know, you tell me. Are they?"

"Of course. I wouldn't be in business if they weren't."

I buried my face in my hands. "That makes it worse!" I wailed. "If everyone else is struggling like this, why can *they* still go out to the bar after work or on weekend trips with their friends or even just to the gym every night? How do they even *have* friends? When I try to do these things, it's like I'm trapped in mud. Strangers ask me what's wrong. I've never seen anyone *else* crying in the bathroom at work because they're burned out by eleven in the morning. And I know, I know, Instagram isn't real life, but all I see are photos of people hanging out with their friends, but when I do it, it all seems like pretend. If everyone else feels like this, I clearly can't even struggle right."

Laura opened her mouth to speak, then closed it, so I barreled on.

"I've seen therapists before and they say it's anxiety, it's depression, it's ingratitude, it's a blocked heart chakra. I've been on Wellbutrin and Lexapro and Prozac, and they all make me feel *wrong*. I could never fall asleep while on Lexapro; the Prozac made me so numb I couldn't feel anything; and don't get me started on the Wellbutrin. I have these . . . tics, I guess, and the Wellbutrin makes me feel like I'm glitching."

Whenever I thought too hard about it all—the breakup, the move, the new job, the same fucking feelings I'd had since I was a kid—my head crackled with dizziness. Nothing would ever change, I was always going to be like this.

"I wonder . . ." Laura said, then paused, as if searching for the right words.

"What?" I pressed, desperate to hand it all to her, desperate for her to fix me.

"Have you read the book *The Highly Sensitive Person*?"

"No, but I've heard that phrase before."

"What do you know about it?"

"Well." I shifted on the couch. I wanted to tuck my feet under me but wasn't sure if it was allowed. I pulled a pillow into my lap instead and hugged it, fiddling with the piped seam along the edge. "After I graduated college I joined a women's group in New York, and there was this woman, Erin, who kept talking about being 'highly sensitive,' but she seemed kind of cuckoo."

Laura jotted a note on her yellow legal pad. "In what way?"

"Oh, just like she was looking for reasons to be special. It was all like, *I can't sit with the group, I need to be farther away because I'm a highly sensitive person. Or, Can we dim the lights? It's giving me a migraine, I'm a highly sensitive person, you know . . .*"

Laura looked at me for a long moment. "Do you think she was perhaps making accommodations for herself?"

I blinked. *Making . . . accommodations . . .* "What do you mean?"

"Well, for a highly sensitive person who finds being around too many people agitating, sitting away from the group might have allowed her to participate without exceeding her own capacity. I wonder what might have happened had Erin *not* disclosed but sat separate from the group without saying anything."

Huh.

If Erin had dimmed the lights, then sat in the corner by herself, I would have thought she was rude.

"Okay," I conceded. "I see what you're saying. We can't win then, can we?"

"It is unrealistic to expect society will magically accept you overnight, but I think you should read the book. It might help you understand yourself, and then we can figure out how to rearrange your life to make it more manageable. There are many HSP qualities that match up with what I'm hearing from you."

"Like what?" I was dying to know how she saw me.

"Feeling exhausted in a bright, open-plan office after a few hours sounds like sensory overload; crashing in bed to watch TV sounds like needing to retreat to a dark, quiet room after being overstimulated all day; plus, being afraid to make accommodations for yourself makes me wonder whether you were called overly sensitive or maybe even unreasonable as a kid . . ."

I sat up straighter. *Check, check, check.*

Back at the office, I squinted at the fluorescent lights and my colleagues buzzing around the lounge area and wondered whether the world was taking something away from me, rather than the other way around. I immediately bought the book.

That night I crawled into bed to read. The preface included a self-test featuring twenty-three true or false statements. I mentally checked off the ones that resonated:

I am easily overwhelmed by things like bright lights, strong smells, coarse fabrics, or sirens close by.
Other people's moods affect me.
Changes in my life shake me up.
When I must compete or be observed while performing a task, I become so nervous or shaky that I do much worse than I would otherwise.
I find myself needing to withdraw during busy days, into bed or into a darkened room or any place where I can have some privacy and relief from stimulation.
I am particularly sensitive to the effects of caffeine.
I am deeply moved by the arts or music.
When I was a child, my parents or teachers seemed to see me as sensitive or shy.

Lying in the dark, I repeated *true, true, true* to the thrum of my heart. I checked twenty-one out of twenty-three statements. The cutoff for being considered highly sensitive was twelve.

Over the next couple of weeks, I read the book whenever I had a few minutes. Every story from HSPs was like reading an entry from one of my diaries.

Elaine Aron, the author, "hid from the chaos" of her family. She "avoided sports, games, and kids in general."

As a child, one of her clients, named Rob, was afraid of everything: of "pinecones, of figures printed on his bedspread, of shadows on the wall."

A woman named Kristen had a creepily familiar crisis her freshman year of college, after transitioning from her small private high school to an overstimulating campus away from home. She quickly fell in love, then traveled to Japan to meet her boyfriend's family. "It was while she was in Japan that, in her words, she 'flipped out.' Kristen had never thought of herself as an anxious person, but in Japan, she was overcome by fears and could not sleep. Then she became depressed. Frightened by her own emotions, her self-confidence plummeted. Her young boyfriend could not cope with her 'craziness' and wanted to end the relationship."

Recognition raced through me. I had always been a balloon, floating above everyone, and someone had just grabbed the string and pulled me back to earth.

With Laura's help, we made small changes to the way I lived and worked and socialized. I splurged on a pair of noise-canceling headphones and a subscription to Spotify. The moment I sat at my desk I popped in my headphones and played white noise all day. The sound dampened my quivering nerves and had the remarkable side effect of limiting how many coworkers approached me. At night, I declined social invitations without (much) guilt. I understood why I'd never like that sort of thing. I still yearned for friendship, so I invited a few coworkers over to my apartment for a casual dinner. Life was starting to feel a little lighter, a little quieter.

A few months later, at the height of foggy San Francisco summer, my office hosted a mandatory team-bonding camping trip at the American River. Laura and I decided that I'd set some boundaries ahead of time so I wouldn't feel so self-conscious bowing out when I started to get overstimulated. Before we left, I summoned the courage to tell Caroline, our office manager and de facto people wrangler, that I didn't do well socializing for long periods of time and likely wouldn't be able to participate in every activity. My hope was that if I preemptively shared this information, I'd feel less shitty about myself when I shut down in the middle of dinner.

"It's a *team*-bonding trip," Caroline reminded me, eyes locked on her computer, while I hovered nervously in front of her desk.

"Yes, of course, I know," I said, flustered. "I just wanted to warn you."

"Okay." She didn't seem too bothered, or maybe I'd made a social error by bringing it up, like Erin from my New York women's group. I slunk away and hoped the trip would go more smoothly.

The night of our work retreat, my coworkers congregated around the fire in a mismatched collection of camp chairs. Macklemore blasted on our CEO's Bluetooth speakers. Everyone was laughing and screaming and telling stories, opening beer bottles, breaking the occasional wineglass, while the fire cracked and spit. My cheeks twitched and shook as I strained to pull them into an expression that conveyed pleasure, but my lips didn't want to lift. Laura's voice somewhere in the recesses of my brain whispered, *It's okay to ask for what you need.*

I walked over to Caroline, who was chatting with a small group.

"Hey, I'm so sorry," I said, touching her lightly on the arm. "I've hit my wall. I need to go to bed."

Caroline rolled her eyes so hard I worried they'd get stuck in her brain.

"Okay, Marian," she snapped. "You've told us a million times. We get it. Go back to your tent."

I did as I was told, but the joy of snuggling up in my sleeping bag with a good novel had vanished. My book remained unopened, perched on my stomach, rising and falling as I tried not to cry. I stared at the slippery gray ceiling of the tent and listened to their distant laughter through the thin plastic.

YEARS EARLIER, WHEN I was eighteen, I took the Myers-Briggs test, a personality type indicator created in the 1940s. My result was INFJ—introverted, intuitive, feeling, and judging—but it was the word *introverted* that resonated with me most. I learned about introversion and immediately understood that, yes, I was quiet and reserved and antisocial, but so was nearly half the population. For a while, *introverted* was enough to explain me to myself.

Highly sensitive was the next phrase I discovered. I wasn't just introverted, but *overstimulated*.

Did *highly sensitive* answer every question I'd ever had about myself? Did it explain my near-constant social faux pas, my brusqueness, my tics, my deep but fleeting obsessions? No, but it explained my overwhelm, and when I was twenty-five, nothing else had come close to capturing how it felt to exist in my body. Another small piece of the puzzle of myself had fallen into place.

Nearly every late-diagnosed autistic person I've spoken with had this same experience: before getting diagnosed with autism, we latched on to the phrase *highly sensitive*.

Like Kristen Hovet, host of *The Other Autism* podcast. Kristen discovered Elaine Aron's work in her late twenties. "I immediately felt like I'd found a way to describe myself and my challenges," she told me. She read and highlighted and reread the book. She did the worksheets and had all her friends complete the assessments too.

Ten years later, Kristen was diagnosed autistic.

The more she learned about how often autistic women are missed as children, and the ableist ways we as a society try to avoid using the word *autism*, the more she realized high sensitivity and autism were likely one and the same. She wrote a powerful opinion piece on Medium on the subject.

"The description of someone who is Highly Sensitive sounds a lot like the description of what was formerly known as 'high functioning autism' or 'Asperger syndrome.' . . . The checklists for women on the spectrum . . . overlap on every single one of the 27 HSP checklist items."

Elaine Aron coined the term *highly sensitive* in the 1990s—a decade when autism was a terrifying concept for parents, and euphemistic phrases like *indigo child* were all the rage. *Highly sensitive* became a more palatable way to talk about developmental disorders.

Enough people have wondered whether there's a link between autism and HSP that Dr. Aron created a page on her website to address whether her definition of sensitivity differed from the official definition of autism. "No one who loves a child or their parents would want to think about autism," she wrote, "even when the child in question will eat only exactly three kinds of food or is happy for twenty minutes merely watching a bicycle wheel spinning."

She insisted the two were separate, basing that belief on *Rain Man* stereotypes of autistic people as incapable of empathy or creativity. Yet Aron herself admitted that the grandnephews she'd previously identified as highly sensitive were, in fact, diagnosed autistic years later. Her team has since deleted this response on her website and replaced it with a simple "This area is not Elaine's specialty, and she does not keep up on current research."

Don't get me wrong: the HSP label has helped countless people, especially women. The label helped me, for a while. It got me 10 percent of the way there—10 percent happier, 10 percent more attuned to my body's responses to the world, 10 percent closer to knowing myself. The concept opened my eyes, for a second, to a glimmer of hope that I was designed this way and that the core of who I am might not need to be fixed but embraced.

HSPs were curious, emotionally sensitive, and able to identify patterns mere normies could only dream of. "You were born to be among the advisors and thinkers, the spiritual and moral leaders of your society," Aron wrote. "There is every reason for pride."

More than twenty years later, *The Highly Sensitive Person* has sold nearly a million copies, birthing its own cottage industry. Aron has published companion workbooks and survival guides and spin-off books about the highly sensitive child and the highly sensitive parent and how to be highly sensitive in love. You can hire a certified coach or take an uncertified online program to learn "sensory-friendly self-care that will help you access your unique gifts."

The problem is, HSP isn't a formal diagnosis. It's not in the *DSM-5*, and there's no official screening process—which means identifying as an HSP is purely personal and won't give you protections should you need them. When I asked Kristen Hovet how her autism diagnosis benefited her more than the HSP label, she told me, "Here in Canada, you cannot get accommodations by saying you're an HSP. Like, good luck with that. But with my autism diagnosis, I was able to partner with my boss to figure out accommodations that allow me to work almost entirely from home."

Then there's the medical impact. Many autistic folks have co-occurring health conditions like epilepsy, colitis, cardiomyopathy, sleep disorders, and Ehlers-Danlos syndrome. "Doctors are aware of these connections," Kristen said, "so if you go into their office with an autism diagnosis, they'll be more likely to look out for these conditions. If you start going on about being an HSP, they're not going to make the connection and will probably dismiss you completely."

Now, is every person who identifies as HSP actually autistic? Maybe not, but it seems likely they're neurodivergent—with diagnosable conditions like ADHD or OCD. Today, some therapists acknowledge this, using *highly sensitive* and *neurodivergent* interchangeably, but that wasn't my experience, and Dr. Aron's book doesn't use the term *neurodivergent* at all. I worry that the HSP label prevents many women from getting a proper diagnosis. When Kristen found out she was autistic at thirty-nine, she got whole body chills.

I don't blame Laura or Dr. Aron or any of the other therapists or self-help programs or books or meditation apps I tried to fix the things about me that were really just neurodivergence. These were the tools available based on passed-down knowledge. Depressingly little research has been done on autistic girls, so why would it have occurred to any of them that the desperate, fidgeting women begging on their couches weren't merely sensitive but something else entirely?

—12—

First Sight

THE DAY I MET MY HUSBAND, I SNUCK OUT OF WORK EARLY. IT WAS four o'clock on a Thursday, my boss was in a meeting downstairs, and the dark loft of our office was empty and quiet. My gut told me to slink out the door before anyone noticed I was gone.

I'd been on a million lackluster OkCupid dates since arriving back in the States; I knew this one shouldn't be any different, but my hands shook as I drove home. I ran up the stairs to my third-floor apartment two at a time. I flung off my jeans and grabbed the outfit I'd laid out that morning: a colorful patterned miniskirt, a white T-shirt, and tall leather boots. I pulled them on and tried to calm down.

Elliot and I had been talking since Sunday. I'd messaged him, attracted to his shamelessly nerdy profile, which listed "tide pooling" as his main interest, along with building Lego ("You'll either find this dorky or endearing," he wrote) and sewing handmade quilts with his mom. After months of weeding through profiles featuring the tedious trifecta of "travel-hustle-sports" topped with unsmiling shirtless selfies, the earnest candor in Elliot's unselfconscious, grinning photos was a shining lighthouse flashing my name.

I sent him a quick message. I'm going to go with endearing re: Lego set. Though it was really the quilt story that won me over.

He replied within the hour. Yea, it's a pretty awesome quilt with sharks on it. You'd be impressed with the craftsmanship if you saw it. Though I do have to admit that my mom did help me finish it.

I sat in bed for hours that afternoon toggling between our increasingly novel-length messages and episodes of *Game of Thrones*. We talked about the places we'd traveled and where to find the best coffee in San Francisco. Then he suggested, "I think we should get coffee and buy you a Lego set sometime. What do you think?"

I was ten minutes early to our first date at Four Barrel Coffee, an industrial, wooden, Edison-bulb-lit monstrosity on Valencia Street, so I ordered a decaf latte and snagged two seats at the high top overlooking the front patio.

When Elliot walked in, I recognized him immediately. He looked exactly like his profile, with deep-set dark eyes underneath thick eyebrows, on a boyish face. My face heated up like the mercury in a thermometer in an old-timey cartoon.

We fumbled as we tried to shake hands, then he was gone again to order his coffee. I sat there hyperventilating.

I'm not a spiritual person. I don't believe the universe has our backs. I don't believe in soulmates. Hell, I barely believe in dietary supplements. But on this day, June 13, 2013, I met a man in a coffee shop and something deep inside me shook loose, as if my very bones were trying to escape. It was warm in the café, my calves sweating in my boots, yet I shivered like I was trapped in a blizzard.

We talked nonstop for the next hour. He was from the Bay Area. No, he didn't have siblings. Well, he used to. His brother, Casey, had died a few years earlier. He lived in the Marina with two friends from high school, and he laughed that the neighborhood wasn't really on-brand for him, given the majority population of white frat boys and streets that flowed with bottomless mimosas. He hadn't traveled much, but he'd gone scuba diving in Honduras and couch surfing in St. Thomas. He asked questions about where I'd lived, what I did for work. He was curious about my writing and acted like it was the coolest job in the world.

I barely understood what he did—something to do with solar panels and engineering and electricity. I spent most of our date staring at his forearms. He wore a navy-blue cardigan over a white button-down. Peeking out a quarter inch from his right sleeve was the blue tip of a tattooed star. That was all I could focus on. That blue star and the tendon in his wrist and the smattering of dark hair and the movement of muscle as he readjusted his grip on his coffee cup. There was a whole universe in that forearm. I was practically panting.

Drinks drained, scone picked apart and abandoned in a pile of crumbs, we walked outside and stopped at a blue Italian scooter that was, apparently, his. He showed it off like a toddler with a crayon drawing, and I melted at the vulnerability of him.

"Can I get your number?" he asked, helmet tucked under his arm.

"Of course." I fumbled for my phone, nearly dropping it on the street.

On the drive back to my apartment, I wondered how many days it would be before I heard from him again, if I did at all.

Twenty minutes later my phone pinged.

Do you want to go for a hike this weekend?

We texted the entire next day, mostly jokes. My cheeks hurt from laughing.

That Saturday he picked me up at seven in the morning in his roommate's beat-up Honda CR-V.

"Where exactly are we going?" I asked, buckling my seat belt.

All he'd told me was that we were taking his favorite waterfall hike, but I didn't know exactly where it was. He might be driving us far out of the city so he could murder me in the woods and wear my skin like a little hat, but my brain was not the organ making the decisions.

"Fairfax," he said, looking over his shoulder.

He placed his hand on the headrest of the passenger seat and backed smoothly out of the driveway. Oh god, his forearm was *right by my face*! Why is that move so sexy? When I drive in reverse, my eyes dart in every direction like a little creature about to scamper into the underbrush, while I'm also somehow hunched over the steering wheel like a geriatric, hands exactly at ten and two. A geriatric scampering into the underbrush: that's me trying to drive in reverse.

Forty minutes later we were in Fairfax, a quirky town that's 70 percent redwood tree, 30 percent crystal emporium. The air itself smells of incense.

We pulled up to a small hiking trail and stepped over ferns peeking out from mossy rocks and through stretches of towering redwoods, their craning necks disappearing into collars of green needles. Under the canopy it was dry and woody, and the familiarity of it comforted me, as if I'd already lived this day with him.

It was too dry for waterfalls, and my perfect bouncing ponytail wilted in the heat. Elliot led me up another switchback. I was going to die. Whenever we got to a reasonably flat section we talked—so fast neither of us could really keep up. Once he'd shaken off his shyness, he told me about a pair of sugar gliders he had after college; his best friend Ben, with whom he now lived; his complicated feelings about his brother's death. He was so *unselfconscious*. I was used to men being mostly interchangeable—every boyfriend I'd had watched sports, drank beer, and wanted a girlfriend who was cool but still girly, available but never clingy.

Elliot did none of those things. He was weird but with such confidence that being around him made me want to reveal my own weird self.

For a while I hid my wheezing, trying to seem more in shape than I really was, until finally I admitted, "Dude, I'm going to die, I cannot keep up with you." And he laughed and hung back, and we sat on a rock while I chugged from my water bottle and fixed my ponytail.

We turned around before we got to the top, hungry and eager for lunch. He led me to a café downtown where we ate chicken salads and talked some more. I don't think there was a minute of silence in the eight hours we spent together that day. I wasn't scared of silence with him; I just had so much to tell him, like we were old friends catching up after twenty years apart.

After lunch, we walked back to the car, and as we crossed the street, he grabbed my hand and interlaced his fingers through mine. I looked at our clasped hands, then at him. My heart became a red-wood tree, too wide around for my chest to contain.

"Hi," I said with a surprised smile.

"Hi," he said back.

We held hands the whole drive home.

I didn't have to guess whether he liked me, I could see it. His face was the clearest face I'd ever seen. His emotions were almost exaggerated, like those charts you see in preschool classrooms that say "Surprised" and "Happy." I could read him like I read my books, his character motivations just legible words on a page rather than a pantomime requiring the constant guessing and adapting I had to do with everyone else.

When we pulled up to my apartment, he parked and walked me to the front door. Would he kiss me? Should *I* kiss *him*?

It was maybe five steps. It took twelve years.

I turned around to say goodbye, but I didn't have the chance to speak before he tugged me to him. I was flooded with so much bliss that it almost edged into despair. It was familiar and brand-new. Some part of my body was being physically soldered onto his.

I heard the sigh of the twenty-three bus across the street and wondered for a moment whether anyone could see us. And then I didn't care at all.

ELLIOT TEXTED ME THE next morning.

> Is it crazy if we have another date tonight?

I was at brunch with Chelsea, who'd moved to San Francisco around the same time as I had. We hadn't seen each other in years, having grown apart in the way childhood friends do, but she bounced out of her seat when I relayed every detail of my date with Elliot. "Should I wait?" I asked her. "Play it cool?" We both agreed that was stupid.

NOT CRAZY, I scream-texted back to him. LET'S DO IT.

We went out for Mexican food that very night and came back to my apartment to "watch a movie." We didn't even make it to the opening sequence. Instead, we sat on the living room couch and made out between progressively deeper conversations about our beliefs and our desires in a partner.

"Abortion?"

"Pro."

"Politics?"

"Blue."

"Children?"

"Yes. Maybe? Someday?"

"Career?"

"Meh. Means to end."

"Travel?"

"YES. Endless. Where do we go first?"

"Monogamy?"

"Ideally."

"I just don't want to pretend to be someone I'm not," I told him.

"Me neither. Let's just skip that part."

He slept over that night. The next morning, without discussing it, we both quietly deleted our OkCupid profiles.

My Facebook messages, Google Chat, and texts during this time were out of control. We were possessed, and we knew exactly what was happening as it was happening, the mad obsession of new love without any of the agony. In one series of escalating messages, Elliot texted me:

> I KEEP LOOKING AT YOUR PHOTOS AND SMILING
> this has seriously never happened to me before
> I've never been so obsessed with looking at pictures of myself with a girlfriend
> IS THAT WEIRD?
> I WANT TO PRINT OUT THE PICTURES OF YOU AND ME AND WALK AROUND MY OFFICE AND SLAP PEOPLE IN THE FACE WITH THEM WHILE SAYING "LOOK AT THESE! LOOK HOW CUTE WE ARE!!! LOOK!!! LOOK!!"

When I wasn't around him, I couldn't think about anything else.

At the two-week mark he messaged me, I have something I need to tell you tonight while giving you five minutes of uninterrupted eye contact.

"I'm kinda sorta falling in love with you," he told me later as we lay in bed facing each other.

"Kinda sorta?" I responded, eyebrows raised. "Try that again."

"I am *absolutely* in love with you."

The world was a sparkling magical place. No amount of time with him was enough. I'd never been in a relationship like this, one so comfortable, one where I knew exactly where I stood.

After years of trying to guess and pretend my way through relationships, Elliot was a well-worn path through dense woods. The only place I'd ever felt at home.

TWO MONTHS AFTER WE met, I moved out of my dreamy sublet in Noe Valley and into his shared apartment in the Marina.

"We know where this is going," he told me when I hemmed and hawed about getting my own place first. The only guy I'd ever lived with before was Lewis. "Why wait?"

Every night after work we ran home, crawled into bed, and stared at each other.

Eye contact has never been my favorite thing. It's a physical discomfort, like a bra strap digging into your shoulder or a small rock in your shoe. Something is just *wrong*.

If my hand were to brush a hot stove, my body would yank away. I don't sit around analyzing *why*, my body just does it. The same is true for eye contact. My reflex is, always, to pull away. I can hold it for a little while, but the whole time I'm thinking about when I can stop.

So when Elliot half-jokingly said, "Let's go home and stare at each other!" I can't pretend a flutter of dread didn't swoop through my belly. Just a small one. Not enough to think more about it. And he looked at me with such tenderness in his dark, deep-set eyes. "Kind eyes," I've heard them called. His hand rested on my hip, rubbing the skin on my side with his thumb, eyes gazing into mine.

"You have such a good face," he said.

Two thoughts jostled inside me. At first I thought, *I love him so much. How is it possible to love someone this much?*

Then another thought, just a flicker in the back of my head: *When can I look away? If I look at his ear, will he still think I'm participating?*

My eyes filled with unwanted tears and I felt myself start to shake. I jolted up in bed and mumbled, "I'll be right back."

I ran into the bathroom and slid against the closed door until I was sitting on the damp tile and cried like he was going off to war.

He doesn't know the real you, he's going to leave, everyone leaves, this relationship isn't real, you can't keep up this lie.

I wailed and wailed, stifling the sounds in my hands so he couldn't hear. (Our bathroom was right next to the bedroom. There was no way he missed this.)

Eventually, when the hiccuping stopped and I was wrung out on the bathroom floor, I padded back to our room, where he was lying starfished on the bed and looking at the ceiling.

"What's going on?" he asked.

The tears threatened to come again, and I pressed my lips together and opened my eyes wide to keep them inside.

"I'm waiting for you to see the real me and realize you don't actually love me and that you want to leave."

He shuffled over to make room and patted the mattress next to him. "Come here."

I crawled back into my side of the bed and he wrapped his arms around me and pulled me close.

"You have nothing to worry about. I love you so so so so much. I'm not going anywhere."

"But how do you *know* that? You can't possibly know that. You say that now but—"

"I just do." He shrugged. It was simple for him. Uncomplicated. It took no more thought than that.

I still didn't believe him. How could I? He thought he knew me now, but eventually he would find out I was crazy, friendless, unpleasant, lazy, weird. He'd pull away and wonder where the fun Marian who hiked and traveled the world had gone. I knew I couldn't sustain the charade forever, and so I ran to the bathroom and cried, once a week, for months.

He didn't leave.

When I suspected that he might really stay, I revealed myself in hushed nighttime conversations—about being an HSP, and about how hard I found it to work in a bustling office, about Chelsea and Elena, about tattling on the kids in Spain, about feeling left out in a family of brothers, about Lewis and his parents in New Zealand, about Ami's journal.

And even then, he didn't leave.

IN EARLY FALL 2013, Elliot and I purchased a baby-blue miniature chalkboard at the Treasure Island Flea Market and hung it on our bedroom wall. Every morning before work, one of us would write a love note to the other. *You're the best*, he wrote. *I fucking love you*, I wrote back. We called it our Chalkboard of Romance.

> *Nice ass.*
> *Have a great day at work!*
> *I like your face.*

One evening in October, I met him in North Beach at an unassuming café that served New Zealand flat whites, then he took me to browse the travel section at City Lights bookstore. Afterward, we stumbled back to our apartment, giddy and holding hands. The house was dark, which meant our roommates were probably out, but we'd apparently left the lights on in our bedroom, because a warm glow was leaking through the cracks around the door. He looked back at me, smiled, then pushed the door open.

Our bedroom was full of candles. Candles on the long, low dresser we'd just bought from IKEA. Candles covering the bedside tables. Candles on the bookshelf. Candles on the small ledge of our chalkboard, which now read:

> *Marry me?*

Elliot grabbed my hands in his. He looked nervous, but his voice was steady.

"You know how much I love you," he said.

Any beautiful and romantic words I wanted to say back caught in my throat and instead I simply said, a little too loud, "Holy shit."

I did know how much he loved me. With Elliot, I could be both the best and the truest version of myself, stripped of everyone I'd ever tried to be. Even though I didn't have a word yet for who I was, Elliot saw her anyway and loved me not in spite of, but because.

He reached behind his back to grab a small wooden box from the chalkboard ledge, then popped it open with one hand. Inside was a simple white gold ring with a small princess diamond in the center.

"Will you marry me?"

Of course I said yes.

The next October, Elliot and I married in the backyard of an Airbnb down the street from our apartment. We didn't tour a million venues or taste seventy-five cakes. We found cheap decorations on Amazon, bought flowers from a street cart, got two simple celebration cakes from a local bakery, and ordered our outfits online. In attendance were thirty people, and we fed them takeout from our favorite restaurant.

After walking each other down the aisle, partners going in and coming out, I stood across from him in view of our families and a smattering of friends. I've always hated birthdays; with everyone's eyes on me as they sing, I feel like I have to perform enjoyment. Getting married felt a little like that, with thirty pairs of eyes on me, watching my reaction to see if I demonstrated love right. The sun beat too hot on my skin, my hands were sweaty in Elliot's hands, I didn't know where to look, but his gaze was steady on me while I looked at the edges of him—the soft lobe of his ear, a thick eyebrow, the dusting of gray at his temples, the crinkles next to his eyes. Our audience disappeared. It was just me and him, tying ourselves together exactly as we were.

That night we took a shared Uber to a karaoke bar. Instead of a first dance we had rehearsed a first song: "A Whole New World" from Disney's *Aladdin*, which we'd practiced together every night on our queen bed. We nailed it.

Around midnight, I couldn't keep my eyes open a second longer. I wanted to be done. I was happy, but weary and sweaty and eager to be alone with Elliot in our cozy studio apartment.

"Can we go?" I asked him even as I thought, *Can you do that? Just leave your own wedding?*

"Absolutely," he said.

We hugged our guests goodbye. "I've never seen you so happy," they told me. "You look so *free*."

When we got back to our apartment, Elliot and I stood together in the kitchen, wrapping a piece of wedding cake in layers of tinfoil to save for our first anniversary. Midwrap he grabbed me by the shoulders and said quietly, "I love you so much, you have no idea." We stood there, hips bumped up against the kitchen island, and breathed into each other. I still can't believe how lucky I am.

—13—

A Little Bit Autistic

I HAD TO GET OUT OF THE OFFICE. EVERY ATOM IN MY BODY SHRIEKED, *Home!* The siren song vibrated my bones and raked down my skin. Would I make it out of the building, or would I simply collapse in the corner of the lobby, hoping for someone to scoop me up and pour me into bed?

At 5 p.m., I fled. An hour in stop-and-go traffic, over the Golden Gate Bridge, off exit 445, racing through yellow lights, instant turns on red, and finally finally finally finally to our new apartment, a granny flat outside San Francisco to which we'd moved shortly after our wedding, glowing like a beacon above the garage.

Once I unlocked the heavy wooden door, Homer, our fluffy white Samoyed, thumped his tail against the couch. For a minute I let him climb all over me, but I couldn't take any more need, any more demands. I was starving, but I couldn't continue standing upright, so I let Homer outside and crawled into bed, wrapping the heavy gray duvet around me until I was an overstuffed burrito. *It's not enough.* I wanted to sink completely into the mattress, let it swallow me whole.

Homer scratched at the door to be let in. A choked wail escaped my throat.

He scratched again.

I huffed, then spent a minute untangling myself from the duvet, stomped over to the door and flung it open before slamming it shut the second he trotted inside, happily bumping the crease of my knee with his wet nose. I hated him.

I climbed back into bed and rewrapped myself. *Still not enough.*

The front door clicked open, and I sighed in relief.

"Hey, babe!" Elliot called out.

"In here." My voice was muffled through the blankets.

From my cocoon I heard Elliot's bag drop and the rustling of his shoes and jacket, then footsteps padding over.

"You okay?"

"No." I said. "I'm feeling a little bit autistic."

"Do you want me to lie on you?"

"Yes please."

I opened the duvet and unfurled myself. Elliot climbed into bed next to me, then draped his entire body on top of mine. The air rushed out of my lungs in one big heave, and with it, the open-plan office and the fluorescent lights and the honking cars and the constant conversation and the traffic and the endless, pointless meetings. The itchy feeling that had spread along my skin was extinguished. I felt whole again.

I don't remember the first time I asked Elliot to lie on me like that, or what made me think it would help. I used the word *autistic* as a stupid joke, long before I was diagnosed, but now I wonder whether my body understood something my brain couldn't. I knew nothing about autism then, but I knew enough about my skin to ask for the pressure.

By twenty-seven I hadn't managed to keep a job for more than a year. I'd quit or been fired from restaurants and temp agencies and law offices, from jewelry stores and art galleries, from jobs as a researcher and hotel housekeeper and cupcake icer and publicity assistant.

The publicity gig was my first big-girl job after college, and in the recession, I was grateful to be employed anywhere. Around the four-month mark, my boss, Edith, greeted me one morning with a stack of printed pages—my work emails. She'd highlighted the parts that were "unprofessional" and lectured me in front of the entire office about appropriate tone.

A week later, I quit and got a job working in the gift shop at the Museum of Sex on Fifth Avenue, where I lasted three months before getting fired for not smiling enough.

"I can't force myself to smile," I told the supervisor, whose name I've long since forgotten.

"Well then," she said, "sounds like you have a choice to make. Either act more pleasant around our guests or leave."

I left.

No one seemed to understand—it *wasn't* a choice. I couldn't force my face to look the way everyone wanted it to look. I can no more smile while overstimulated than I can jump off my roof and fly into space. When surrounded by stimuli, the vestigial aspects of my personality shut down, as if going into power-saving mode. Until I'm fully charged, those features are offline.

Near the end of my time at Couchsurfing, which lasted a whopping eleven months, my boss, Mel, invited me to a daylong working retreat at the CEO's glossy SoMa apartment. In attendance would be the three department heads—of marketing, product, and engineering—along with the CEO. It didn't make any sense, I was a low-level marketing manager: Why would they want me there? After thinking about it for a day, I figured that if I'd been invited it meant I'd proven my value. *They must want me for my big, brilliant brain!*

On the day of the retreat, motivated by Mel's confidence in me, I was *on fire*. I listened thoughtfully. I asked pointed questions. When the VP of product started arguing with the VP of engineering about missed deadlines, I asked, "Why exactly won't this be ready in time?" If I could understand the delay, I could help solve it. Once they explained the two competing priorities, I said, "Well, from what I see on social, 80 percent of users say they want a calendar, so let's hold off on Place Pages and knock the calendar out in a three-week sprint."

Man, I was brilliant. *Irreplaceable.* My work style was unique and, at the right company, could probably form the backbone for a real career.

The next day Mel pulled me aside between our desks.

"Your behavior yesterday was incredibly inappropriate," she said.

My face fell, but I tried to keep my voice emotionless and professional. "How do you mean?"

"Everyone said you were aggressive."

"Wait, *aggressive*? How?"

"Well, *I* didn't think you were aggressive," Mel said, always eager to be the cool boss. "I know that's just how you are, but everyone else was really put off. Your questions came across as rude. You need to apologize."

I ached to defend myself, but I didn't want to come across as *more* aggressive, so I kept my mouth shut and wrote an apology email to the CEO and his triad of VPs.

If you'd asked me to describe my behavior at the CEO's live-edge dining room table, I would have used words like *engaged, thoughtful,* maybe *a little intense* . . . but *aggressive? Rude? Inappropriate?* Like nine-year-old Marian hiding in the woods, I clearly didn't know myself at all.

Still, *autism* wasn't the word that popped into my head. I'd just read *Lean In,* so I assumed I was being judged more harshly for the same behavior men got away with all the time. I blamed my difficulties on the patriarchy, not neurodivergence.

After a mass layoff at Couchsurfing that left me more relieved than crushed, I landed a job at another start-up that boasted three catered meals a day, rooftop yoga, and free monthly massages. I always interviewed well, so getting a new job wasn't hard; I just had a hard time keeping it.

My new office building was open from the ground floor to the fourth—"To keep our creativity flowing," said the young, bearded CEO. There wasn't a single rug or curtain, just hardwood, steel, and glass. You could hear each and every sound that each and every human made in that building: the chatter of customer support; the loud, bro-ey laughter from the sales department; the blenders and timers and food processors in the kitchen. I was on the second floor, sandwiched between it all.

Every day was the same. For the first couple of hours, I was a machine, racing through my checklist, knocking back tasks, but every few minutes, even with my headphones blasting Brown Noise Playlist #3, someone new walked into the building and the thud of the door vibrated up to my desk. As my coworkers thundered in, I waved hello and answered questions. The sounds and interruptions chipped away at my capacity until there was nothing left.

By 11 a.m., the words on my screen blurred. I could no longer piece them into any coherent meaning. While I'd finished the bulk of my work, there were still hours left in the day. I should get ahead, right? The expectations were never clear to me, beyond that I must remain in this building until five o'clock. The thought of this discomfort lasting six more hours fell like a boulder on my back.

This was when I'd sprint to the bathroom. Whenever I feel overwhelmed, I instinctively retreat to small, dark places—the only reliable way I can lower the volume on the world and hear myself think, like my own private sensory deprivation tank.

Most days, I locked the door to the bathroom and sat on the floor, my back slunk against the cool gray tiles. I closed my eyes and focused on my breath.

I imagined inhaling productive energy, filling my lungs with the strength to get through the day. I noticed the tile, cool at my back and under my legs. I lay my hands in my lap, palms up to receive (or was it palms down to ground me? I flipped them back over).

Footsteps outside the bathroom jolted me out of my meditation.

How long had I been in here? What if someone thought I was poop-
ing? I shot up and rushed back to my desk, took another hitching
breath, and looked at my Google Doc again.

The words still swam, digital minnows darting across the screen.
Shit.

It was only 11:10.

I needed fresh air and exercise. That's what the research said,
right? Going outside boosts your energy? Exercise makes you more
productive?

Outside, I took great gulps of air choked with exhaust, hungry
for even the faintest whiff of redwood that sometimes blew in from
the Presidio. Instead, I caught notes of urine, weed, and sweat. Construction clattered and whirred across the street. A scrawny man
stood naked on the sidewalk, flapping his flaccid penis at no one.
Then, in a flash, he ran into traffic, dodging cars like a game of *Frog-
ger.* At one point he stopped, leaned back on his heels, and raised
his arms to the sky, enjoying the sun while cars screeched to a halt,
horns screaming.

I rushed around the corner, trying to concentrate on the blue
sky and the cool breeze. *Blue sky cool breeze blue sky cool breeze.* I
stepped over a pile of shit. Hopefully a dog's, but knowing SoMa,
probably not.

Ten minutes later, back at the office, I didn't even bother going
back to my desk. I already knew I didn't feel better.

I made a beeline for an empty couch, popped in my headphones,
and opened a guided meditation on my phone. I lay down while the
sound of rain washed away the office and the seething street below.

*You're in a cabin with a roaring fire. A huge cushion is laid in front
of the flames. The fire is warming your toes, your ankles, your calves,
your thighs.*

My breath deepened and slowed. Until I sensed footsteps. I
imagined a coworker looming over me while I looked stupid and
vulnerable, lying on the couch doing deep breathing exercises. My

eyes shot open. It was just Miles, twenty feet away. *Keep breathing. Tune them out. You can control this.* My breath caught as someone else lumbered by.

I looked out at the office, watching my coworkers typing away, squinting at their screens, laughing and perched on each other's desks. They weren't thinking about me; I knew that logically, but I could never quite shake the feeling that anyone, at any time, might pull me aside for a lecture on appropriate workplace behavior. Each new job came with a welcome packet, an onboarding PowerPoint, and the constant dread that I was walking around with metaphorical spinach in my teeth.

Defeated, I turned off the meditation and slunk back to my desk, where I spun around in my chair until 5 p.m.

I lasted like this for nearly a year, frantically trying to cure my overstimulation with more stimulation so that I could keep working like everyone else, then rushing home to drown myself in blankets, my only release 160 pounds of husband Heimlich-ing the stress out of me.

ON ONE NIGHT I hid inside my blanket pile with Elliot on top of me, I mumbled, "I hate my job."

Elliot shifted his weight to lie on his side and look at me. "Oh noooo."

"Yeah." I groaned. "I just—I hate going there, but I can't articulate why in any way that makes sense. The work feels impossible, even though I *know* I'm good at it." Future decades of employment rolled out before me in a void of Vantablack. A pressure tightened inside my chest cavity. This was my *one* responsibility as an adult, and I kept failing. Most people would kill for a San Francisco tech job with friendly people, good pay, and extravagant perks. I was so ungrateful. So *weak.*

"Maybe I'm just not cut out to work in an office," I said. I buried my face in his neck, which smelled like cotton and sandalwood, plus something else so distinctly Elliot that I could find him blind in the woods like a frantic little fox.

My go-to option was to quit, but I hesitated this time. What would I do afterward, get another office job? I'd blown through twelve in five years—I knew the solution did not lie in more of the same.

Around the world, countless undiagnosed autistic people experience similar challenges, chronically underemployed, unable to manage a standard day's work, and lectured for behaviors they don't understand. Like Jenara Nerenberg, a graduate of Harvard, MIT, *and* UC Berkeley. In her midtwenties, Jenara was fired from one of her first journalism jobs. After a bout of freelancing, she tried again at a start-up but was fired after six months. A year later she took a low-paying job in a more arts-oriented organization but, again, was fired after a month. Jenara later learned she was both autistic and had ADHD. In her book, *Divergent Mind*, she wrote, "The hardest part throughout the trials of these various jobs was the overwhelming sense of loss, confusion, loneliness, and uselessness I felt. I had zero vocabulary about neurodivergence—and no one else around me had that vocabulary either."

Writer and photographer Kay Lomas also struggled to stay employed before her autism diagnosis. She couldn't understand why work always felt so challenging and would chastise herself for never sticking with a job. "Although I started a new position with the hope and expectation that *this* job would be OK, sooner or later I would start to get *that* feeling again, like I wasn't fitting in or this company environment wasn't for me." She'd try to hold out as long as she could, but she never made it longer than a year. "I once started a job and left after only two days," she wrote in a blog post for the *Mighty*. "The office was chaotic, noisy and disorganized and the social expectations on staff were high for after work drinks, weekly events and social functions."

Jenara, Kay, and I could feel something was off, but we all assumed that something was our brokenness, and not the unchangeable wiring of our brains. The problem wasn't us, but our environment.

It's estimated that 85 percent of college-educated autistic adults are unemployed or underemployed. That number is staggering, but it's also unsurprising. Traditional work environments are often inaccessible to autistic people. There's the sensory nightmare of open-plan offices, retail stores, or restaurant floors. Office politics. Networking. Incessant meetings. Arbitrary rules.

The interview process alone is a massive barrier to employment. The first thirty seconds require juggling eye contact, social cues, and vague questions with double meanings. Ludmila Praslova, professor of organizational psychology at Vanguard University and late-diagnosed autistic, wrote in *Harvard Business Review*, "The personality-focused job application process is a barrier for many people who may be better at performing the job than at talking about themselves—and it is just one example of the many workplace 'norms' that are not inclusive of neurodiversity."

For masked autistics like yours truly, the interview is the easy part. I'm so adept at mirroring that, for one hour, I can appear the most confident, charming, qualified candidate on the market. When I land an interview, I get hired; but only because every laugh, every smile, every movement is a lie. It's a song and dance I've memorized, but performing for an hour is one thing; it's another thing entirely to maintain the ceaseless choreography for eight hours a day, five days a week. By day two, I'm no longer able to pull on my leotard and tap shoes. It's only a matter of time before I get fired or quit for not being able to sustain the movements I originally promised I could do.

Special education teacher Hyacinth knows this all too well. "I had a job interview today," she wrote in a subreddit for autistic women. "It went great! Can't wait to show up for my first day there as well functioning as a sack full of badgers, ask stupid questions and just silently freak out that I don't already know every routine at the place. I will then throw myself into the job for about a year and then burn out spectacularly. Gonna be a fun ride!"

It's a shame, because, with the right accommodations, autistic people make excellent employees. We have incredible attention to detail and pattern recognition. We're creative problem solvers and can focus for long stretches of time. To resolve this incongruence between our abilities and our opportunities, the Frist Center for Autism and Innovation was founded at Vanderbilt in 2018 with a mission to create pipelines to employment for autistic adults. Director Keivan Stassun, the parent of an autistic son, said, "I would not change my son for the world, so I will change the world for him."

For Keivan, changing the employment world happens through adjustments in recruitment, hiring, and retention. Because I've always had trouble keeping jobs, and that's the area where I see many other late-diagnosed autistics struggling, I called him to ask how they're working on this.

"I think about retention in two buckets," he said. "One is what we call accommodations and support. These can be simple assistive technologies that allow individuals to remain in an environment that might otherwise be challenging. That can mean noise-canceling headphones or access to a quiet space. It can also mean participating in meetings outside of a traditional conference room—say, in a quiet room in the same building or remotely from home.

"The second bucket is ultimately more important, and it's about the workplace itself. Workplace culture very often revolves around many things that have nothing to do with the actual work, which is where you can have these cultures like the ones you experienced." I had told him about the Couchsurfing camping trip and the Burning Man–themed party the company hosted a month later, where my boss had hotboxed me in a van. "Do they want to be a fraternity?" he said. "Or do they want to be an environment with clear communication and productive workers? One of the most important ways leaders can create inclusive work environments is by making it clear to all managers and employees that what *really* matters is precise communication and quality in work product. The expression on your face and the tone of your language—those things should become secondary."

Today, the Frist Center partners with companies that help create neuroinclusive cultures and with hiring platforms that match employers with neurodiverse talent. They also build assistive technologies like job interview simulators and virtual reality–based driving instruction systems. "Only about a quarter of autistic adults are licensed to drive," Keivan told me. "In most places in the US, if you can't drive, it severely limits your options when it comes to work."

These supports can't come fast enough, because most autistic adults aren't working cushy tech jobs with rooftop yoga and three catered meals a day, and those of us who do don't survive long.

OUTSIDE MY DUVET BURRITO, Elliot was still and thoughtful. He knew I craved stability and meaningful work like everybody else. "Could you ask to work from home?" he suggested.

This was 2014. Pre-pandemic, pre-Slack, pre-Zoom. This was the year after Marissa Mayer's leaked Yahoo! memo that banned employees from working from home. As common as remote work is now, the thought hadn't even crossed my mind.

But I was clawing out of my skin, scrabbling at the cage, desperate for relief from the noise and the chaos and the confusion. The next job wouldn't be better, I knew that. I was on a hamster wheel of attrition. I could work from home or quit. I had nothing left to lose.

The next day, before I had the chance to overthink it, I approached my boss, Liam, tentative and stumbling.

"Sure, let's try it," Liam shrugged. He suggested starting with two days a week, then reevaluating.

My productivity skyrocketed. I needed only three to four hours a day to get done what I needed to get done, and without the stimulation of a commute and the distractions of my coworkers, I did my best, most thoughtful work, which made me feel good about myself. By not working in an office, I had fewer chances to offend someone with my blank facial expressions and blunt feedback.

More important, I could breathe again. I lived for those two days—walking Homer at lunchtime, sitting alone at my desk overlooking the pines, the only noise an occasional *thunk* as squirrels dropped acorns on our roof. In those two days a week, when Elliot came home from work, I was cooking or chatting on the phone with a friend or reading on the couch, no longer hiding in a cave made of blankets.

My one-year anniversary at the company came and went, those two days acting as a bolster that supported me through another full year there, the longest I'd ever managed to stay anywhere. I actually *liked* my job. In this small way I learned to stop forcing myself to perform in an environment that wasn't built for me. It was the kindest thing I had ever done for myself.

—14—

Cry Baby

SHE WAS WAILING, BUT I COULDN'T SEE HER.

At least it was a hearty wail. Her lungs clearly worked. I craned my neck to try to see over the blue curtain separating my covered chest from my exposed insides, but it was too tall. All I could see was a wall of blue and all I could hear was Elliot's "*Whoa*," and the doctor explaining somewhere in the distance, "The baby was occiput transverse, meaning oriented to the pelvis . . ." and then Elliot was gone from my side, and I was alone. My body was numb all the way up to my shoulders due to the anesthesia, and I was stuck on the operating table, waiting, listening to her cry.

"Is she okay?" I asked, my voice hoarse after thirty-nine hours of labor. No one answered. I heard her crying kick up a decibel, then the muffled voice of a masked nurse: "Eight pounds, three ounces."

Antiseptic. Alcohol. Wailing. The beep of my heart rate monitor. Blue sheet. Wailing.

Footsteps, rustling, then a warm weight at my shoulder. I turned my head a quarter inch to the right and there she was.

Her little peanut of a body nestled into the crook of my neck, flipped so I could see her face. The warmth of her pressed to the warmth of me. She was wrapped in a pink-and-blue blanket and wore an unfathomably tiny pink hat. Her eyes were round and gray and staring right into mine. I didn't need to look away.

"Hi, June," I whispered. "Hi, sweet girl." Her face relaxed and her crying stopped. For a moment we breathed into each other. *There she is. There's her face. I know that face. That's my daughter.*

I couldn't feel my body, nor the pain from two days of contractions, nor the doctor plopping my insides back in, nor the restitching of my organs and muscle and skin. The surgeon warned I might feel "a little pressure," but I didn't. All I felt was her.

Her pursed lips were full and delicate. Her cheeks were fat, drooping down the sides of her face like pancake batter. Eyelashes dark and wet. Eyebrows straight across her forehead like mine, a baby Frida Kahlo. *Oh my god, is she the most beautiful child who has ever lived? I think she is.* My arms, glued to my sides, ached to touch her, to hold her, to cling her to me.

"I wish I could hold you," I said, my voice breaking.

Thirty minutes later, my arms denumbed, a nurse named April (born in April, unlike June, who was born in May) wheeled me into the recovery room, where my daughter was at last placed into my arms. I was half naked, breasts hanging out for the whole world to see, hair tangled in knots on top of my head. I hadn't slept in days, and the last thing I'd eaten was two days earlier while laughing and doing hip circles on a yoga ball in front of some HBO show about stand-up comedy.

June wiggled like an inchworm and latched on to nurse.

"Hey, this doesn't hurt at all!" I said to Elliot.

He looked on, still wearing scrubs, holding our camera, bags under his eyes, smiling still. The nurses were suspiciously silent. How many new mothers had they seen pass through this room, so in love with our babies that for a few moments we are completely delusional, convinced that the hardest part of parenthood is now behind us?

They say meeting your baby is like nothing you've ever imagined.

You don't know love until you become a parent. You can't possibly understand until it happens to you. Before June was born, I knew I would be the exception. My history of depression and anxiety and therapy and drugs prepared me for postpartum depression, delayed bonding, low milk supply, and regret. I read story after story about women who didn't connect with their babies for the first year. While eight months pregnant, I waddled down our carpeted hallway in the middle of the night to pee for the forty-fifth time, and as I sat there in the dark, my stomach fluttered with her movements and my dread over the inevitable: the moment when I would meet my daughter and feel nothing.

Except that's not what happened.

Motherhood descended upon me like some great winged bird, or an angel, or a ghost at my bedside, hovering above me, waiting for the moment when she could inhabit my skin—the Marian who was a mother becoming one with the Marian who was not.

This tiny, perfect creature was mine, and I was hers, and we had somehow found each other amid the chaos of the universe, and I knew, more than I'd ever known anything in my life, that I could be everything for her. I loved her the way I'd always wanted to be loved—which is to say easily and unconditionally. Loving her was the one thing I had ever done right.

AFTER FOUR DAYS IN the hospital, Elliot, June, and I headed home as a family of three. I rode next to her in the back, where she promptly fell asleep. When we arrived, Elliot carried her, car seat and all, inside the house and placed her on the floor for Homer to greet. He trotted over, gave a quick sniff of her toes, then flopped back down on the couch to gaze out the window.

I sat with him, petting his soft head, waiting for her to wake up. Ten minutes passed, then fifteen. She was still asleep.

I made myself a snack. I heard a rustle and rushed back into the living room, but she'd just moved her foot. I unpacked my hospital bag. I read a book.

Who gets bored with a newborn?

The next two weeks passed in a delicious haze of languid naps and an overabundance of milk. Elliot and I had three months of parental leave, which meant we had nothing to do except enjoy our new daughter and learn how to parent. Every morning Elliot brought me coffee in bed, along with a bowl of yogurt framed by hand-pitted cherries and a drizzle of honey. I ate it as we waited for June to wake up, then I nursed her as the breeze wafted in through the windows and the morning light glinted on dust particles in the air.

At two weeks old, June woke up.

It was 5 a.m., the morning after my parents arrived from Connecticut to meet her. Elliot put her on his chest, where she grunted and wiggled, like she couldn't get comfortable. He tried burping her, patting her back, giving her his finger to suck on.

"Why are you being so fussy?" he asked.

I tensed. *No, everything is perfect, do not acknowledge that any part of this is hard.* And, *So what if she's fussy? Allow her to feel her feelings.*

I took her from him and bounced her up and down. "It's okay, *sh sh sh.* It's okay. Mommy's here." Her grunts became louder. "It's okay, *sh sh sh.*" The grunts turned into wails. Shrieks. I pulled down the top of my nightgown and tried to nurse again. She latched on for a moment, until the milk started flowing too fast and she pulled away, my nipple still in her mouth. Milk sprayed all over her face, down my top and onto the bed.

"Goddamn it," I snapped.

Elliot reached to take her back while I changed my clothes. Then I started yanking the duvet cover off the bed while huffing dramatically. Elliot was bouncing and shushing June, but she was screaming now. The red wail of her caterwauling was like a fire alarm shocking me awake from a deep sleep: jarring and disorienting. It signaled danger. I pressed my hands against my ears and shook it away.

It lasted all day. Elliot and I sniped at each other, passing a screaming June back and forth like a football with a sharp "You take her."

I tried feeding her, changing her diaper, singing, turning the air-conditioning on full blast, the white noise so loud it sounded like we lived inside an airplane hangar. In the afternoon Elliot wrapped her in the carrier and took her and Homer for a walk. Five minutes later he was back, snot dripping down the coffee-colored fabric, June still shrieking.

"Nope. Your turn," he said.

Where had our easy newborn gone? Something had to be wrong. I wondered where I'd put the pediatrician's phone number, then dismissed the thought as I had vowed to never be one of "those mothers." I could handle this myself.

I stripped off her onesie and examined her smooth body for a wasp sting or a deadly rash. Her skin was pristine, except for fresh goose bumps from the air-conditioning. She screamed louder.

"Oh, honey, I'm sorry. I'm so sorry, baby."

I wrapped her in a fresh diaper and soft duck jammies. I pressed her to my chest. I ran through my entire Disney repertoire. I shushed and bounced and sang until my arms threatened to fall off.

The sun was low again over the back fence when at last her cries faded and she fell into a tearstained sleep, starfish-sprawled in the middle of our bed.

Okay, fine. So motherhood wouldn't be as easy as I thought.

JUNE DID NOT STOP crying. She cried on her back in our living room, flailing underneath her play gym, her round belly tensing as she screamed. She cried on our morning walks around the neighborhood while I slumped across the handlebars of her stroller, pushing it up and down the streets of San Rafael, a hopeless Sisyphus.

One evening, in a wishful burst of energy, Elliot and I took her to our local farmers' market. I tucked June into a linen sling across my chest, and the three of us walked downtown. Five minutes later June was wailing, her perfect face scrunched in misery. Across the street, two mothers were walking toward us. One also had her baby in a sling, but her son was quiet and drooling. The other was pushing a stroller, and for a moment I thought it was empty, but no, that baby was sucking on a pacifier, his damp hands gripping a worn blanky, his eyelids fluttering closed. I could hear the women's easy laughter and my stomach roiled with jealousy.

Something *must* be wrong. At June's eight-week wellness check, I explained the myriad ways and places she cried. Our pediatrician, a woman named Francesca who had dark curly hair and a collection of animal-print dresses, nodded. "It sounds like colic to me," she said. "I don't love giving medication to babies, so why don't we try a natural remedy first."

I didn't notice a difference between June with her chamomile drops and June without.

"It could be digestive trouble," Francesca said at our next appointment. "She's older now, so let's try an antacid."

We tried the antacid. Nothing.

At every appointment June was a perfect angel baby, happy and gurgling, while I sobbed on the crinkly paper of the exam room table about how I couldn't handle the noise. During that first year, Francesca eliminated every serious medical condition, and eventually, while it was never explicitly said, the implication was that June's crying was a reflection of our parenting.

There's nothing wrong with her. Babies cry. It's your job to not cater to her so much. She needs to fit into your life, not the other way around.

I read books like *The Explosive Child* and *The Highly Sensitive Child* and *The Whole-Brain Child*. I read the work of Dr. Sears,

Magda Gerber, Ina May, Janet Lansbury. There were manuals for parenting; I just had to follow the instructions, and everything would be okay, right?

The problem was, all the books contradicted each other, and I had no capacity to intuit what was right for *my* child. In the moment, when June was shrieking and I was sleep-deprived and covered in milk, I couldn't remember a thing I'd read. *Am I supposed to let her cry for five minutes before picking her up to see if she self-soothes, or am I supposed to ask permission to pick her up? Will it work as well if it's not skin to skin? But wait, when I touch her, she seems to scream even louder. I must be doing it wrong.*

Francesca said it might just be her temperament, and she would grow out of it when she started talking, but when June was just over a year old and still crying most hours of the day, Francesca referred us to a behavioral psychologist. "June's perfectly healthy," she said, trying to comfort us. "But that doesn't mean there's not something else going on."

To prepare for our appointment with the psychologist, I spent a week working on a document that outlined every behavior.

> She gets extremely anxious in crowds and during periods of transition.
> Terrified to do anything out of our normal routine. In the past month we've tried going on a hike and to a preschool harvest festival, both of which she spent crying until we left.
> Screams any time I leave the room. Seems constantly afraid that I'll leave.
> Tantrums spiral into all-day unhappiness.

We kept trying to take her to farmers' markets and restaurants and seasonal events. Everyone said parenting was hard, but they still managed to take *multiple* children out into the world, so I needed to do that too. If I didn't, I was catering to June's demands, letting a baby call the show. I needed to force her to assimilate, even if it killed us both.

During our first appointment, Elliot and I sat clinging to each other on the sofa across from the psychologist, Dr. Charlotte.

"In cases like these," she said, "it's hard to say for sure what the issue might be. The first thing we usually look at is autism, but I don't think that's what we're dealing with here. She's hit all of her developmental milestones. She may just have some sensory processing issues."

"Wonder where she gets that from." I laughed, though it wasn't funny.

The doctor looked to me. "Are you sensitive?"

"Oh yeah." I laughed again, dry and bitter. "That's one of the reasons this has been so hard. I can't just tune out her crying."

I set up a camera so the doctor could see our daily activities and give her assessment. Dr. Charlotte watched the videos and told me that I "looked anxious" while feeding June her breakfast and that my anxiety was probably rubbing off on her. We talked about attachment issues and how incorporating "consistent positive parenting strategies" might help fix the underlying problems.

For twelve weeks we took June to occupational therapy, where she crawled through soft tubes and was happily pushed on a swing. We found a pediatric chiropractor who charged $150 a session and didn't take insurance. Every week the chiro lay her hands gently on June, while June screamed and I hung back, wincing, trying not to plug my ears or tear out my hair. Nothing gave either of us any relief.

Looking back, this whole time looks eerily similar to my own journey, going from doctor to doctor, *knowing* something was wrong, but given generic solutions and catchall diagnoses, the equivalent of a shrug emoji. And sure, Elliot had a hard time with June's crying too. He was tired and stressed. But the salt in the wound was me, because the whole time June was melting down, so was I.

IT HAPPENED ON A five-minute drive to Walgreens. June was three months old, and I had to grab some ibuprofen. June hated the car and would scream from the second we buckled her in to the second we arrived at our destination and then the entire time *at* the destination. I braced myself for the noise, but when has bracing for pain ever helped you tolerate it?

We backed out of the driveway with a whimper, pulled onto Fourth Street with the first hiccuping cry, and by the halfway mark she was howling, her ferocious shrieks burrowing into my eardrums and latching on with tenacious pinchers.

Every piece of advice I'd read flitted across my field of vision, like those GIFs of geniuses doing complicated math problems, except it was an onslaught of other people's opinions, including respectful parenting and attachment parenting and cry it out and ten thousand other books and podcasts and documentaries.

In this moment I chose what I call "validation jabbering."

The idea is that your child deserves the respect of clear communication, even if you're not going to give in to their demands. You're supposed to validate their feelings, letting them "participate in their own care."

"It's okay, honey, I know you don't like being in the car, we'll get there soon," I said. "Do you want your song? Here, let me turn on your music."

So I was soothing and driving and her wails were getting louder and more piercing and the sound was buzzing through my whole body, threatening to shake my heart straight out of my chest, and I was glancing at my phone trying to find the damn song she liked and when it finally turned on the car was filled with both the gentle sound of the guitar and June's progressively louder screams and I turned into the Walgreens parking lot and *how am I going to grab my ibuprofen when she's like this . . .* and then it all burst out of me, at the full capacity of my lungs.

"SHUT UP SHUT UP SHUT UP JUST SHUT THE FUCK UP! STOP CRYING! I NEED ONE FUCKING FUCK SEC-OND OF SILENCE."

My voice burned up my throat and bounced off the windows. The sound exploded out of the car. Birds scattered somewhere in Wisconsin.

Then for one blissful second, before the shame rushed in, the car and the world were quiet. It took just a moment for June's shock to wear off and then she was wailing again, harder, and this time I joined her, the car filled to the brim with both our tears.

I am a terrible mother. I can't handle even three minutes of crying. I'm not just invalidating her feelings, I'm punishing her for them.

I turned around and drove home without the ibuprofen.

I'd expected postpartum depression, but I hadn't expected this, to love my daughter so fully but be so incapable of being around her for more than a few minutes without losing my mind. I couldn't handle the sensations of motherhood. The constant climbing and pawing. The need to bounce and rock. The crying, the lack of sleep. My body was a too-tight guitar string, ready to snap at any moment. Which I did, at least once a week for two years.

Just before June turned one, we were sitting in the dining room, her in her high chair at the head of the table like some Renaissance lord, me half asleep in the seat next to her.

"Mommy, Baby Shark. Baby Shark!"

"Honey, we listened to 'Baby Shark' seventeen times already. I cannot listen to it anymore."

"Baby Shaaaark!" she whined.

The sound clawed its way into the tubes of my ears and the pain-ful, tender part of my brain. I could barely hear her over the static in my head. My hand twitched. I ached to slam my palms onto the table, to feel the sting of the wood on my skin. Mommy Shark was on her last nerve.

"Baby Shaaaaarrrrkkkk!!!!!"

I closed my eyes. *Focus on your breath.* Inhale, exhale.

"BABY! SHARK!"

I shrunk back, the sound breaking me out of my flimsy meditative state. I must not have taken deep enough breaths.

Just tune it out! I shouted at myself. I remembered Elizabeth Gilbert in *Eat Pray Love* and her successful meditation at an ashram in India even though she was surrounded by biting mosquitoes. "In stillness, I watched myself get eaten by mosquitoes," she wrote. "The itch was maddening at first but eventually it just melded into a general burning feeling and I rode that heat to a mild euphoria."

Where was my euphoria? I closed my eyes again and imagined a bubble surrounding my body, protecting me from the sound. With each inhale, the bubble contracted, and with each exhale, it expanded.

"BABY SHARK BABY SHARK BABY SHARK!!!!!!"

The bubble burst.

Stay calm. Just let her scream. It won't change anything. She has to learn she can't always get what she wants. Remember, your anxiety feeds her anxiety.

I turned to June with my most maternal, empathetic face.

"I know, honey, you really want 'Baby Shark.' You love that song!" As I spoke, the pain in my body twisted somewhere deep. I watched her face crumple and turn red, a dam about to burst, but I kept flailing, grasping for some sense of control over this one-year-old who owned me. I leaned toward her and gently touched her sticky hand where she'd been eating plums from the tree in our backyard. She yanked it away.

"MAMA! BABY! SHARK!"

A Little Less Broken   167

"I know, honey, I know. It's so hard when you can't get what you want."

Each word out of my mouth was fire, but if I couldn't do this, if I couldn't empathize with my daughter who just wanted her favorite song, how the hell would I manage when she was sixteen and I wouldn't buy her a car? *How was I going to do this for seventeen more years?* I forced a smile. She squished the plum in her hand, then smeared it into her hair. Great, now I was going to have to clean it out during bath time, which also made her scream.

On the living room couch, Homer's ears twitched and his head shot up. He barked once, sharp and piercing. I flinched. He bolted to the door and whined.

The doorbell rang.

I groaned and dragged myself from the chair, the smell of plums thick in my nostrils. Homer whined again and ran in circles by the door, his nails clacking like a tap dancer.

I swung open the door. Behind the screen, two older women wearing ankle-length skirts and long-sleeve blouses stood with black leather briefcases and a stack of pamphlets.

Fuck. Jehovah's Witnesses.

"Hello! Good afternoon! My name is Elaine and this is Mary. Can we just—"

I have never in my life been rude to someone at the door; I have let salespeople talk at me for thirty minutes about solar panels and fiber network something-or-others, but not today, Satan.

"I'm sorry," I said tightly, not sorry at all. "I can't with you right now." I slammed the door in their faces.

I walked back to the dining room table with purpose.

"You know what, hun? You wanna listen to 'Baby Shark'? Let's do it." I grabbed my phone and had Spotify open in .3 seconds. The happy notes of "Baby Shark" filled the room.

"NOOOOOOO!!!!" June screamed. She strained against her

high chair, her face the color of plums. I couldn't tell what was fruit and what was anger.

"What is wrong with you?!" I snapped. "You've been begging for 'Baby Shark' for fifteen minutes."

She stiffened and grunted. Her face was turning red. I panicked. Was she choking? In a flash I was unbuckling the straps and lifting her out of her high chair.

"Are you okay, baby? Did something happen?"

She screamed, straining against me now. "Down, Mama! Down!"

"You want to go on the floor?"

"No! Chair!"

"But you were so unhappy in the chair!"

Baby shark do do do do do baby shark do do do do do

"CHAIR!!!! NO BABY SHARK!"

The room spun. Afraid I'd drop her, I put her back in her chair, my lower back spasming as I hunched over, trying to figure out these fucking straps. The song began again, on a hideous loop from hell.

I swung toward my phone and paused the song. June looked at me with her big eyes, tears streaked down her cheeks. I reached over to wipe a bit of juice off her lip, managing only to smear it across her cheek. She looked like a demon.

"BABY . . . SHAAAAAAAARK!!!"

There wasn't a thought that crossed my mind or a moment's hesitation.

I grabbed the empty plum-smeared plate and flung it as hard as I could into the wall.

The thick pottery made a satisfying *CRACK* before breaking into three neat pieces and scattering on the floor.

June's eyes darkened, then her entire face creased. I pounded my hands on the table, then stormed into our bedroom where Elliot was getting ready.

"I threw a plate. I can't do this anymore. Just take her. I can't."

"I got it, don't worry." He rushed out of the room. Behind him, I slammed our bedroom door as hard as I could.

THROWING THE PLATE TOWARD my one-year-old daughter was the worst thing I did, but it also wasn't completely out of character. I smashed two souvenir glasses from a trip to Germany. I slammed more doors more times than I could ever count. I had a lovely, perfect daughter and she was so unlucky to get stuck with me. Though I was thirty-one and married and a mother, I was still twelve inside and full of rage.

After my explosions, I'd run away from June, too ashamed to look at her sweet face. I'd curl up in bed and hide under the blankets until the rage evaporated and my mind cleared.

Hours after throwing the plate, I emerged from the bedroom in surrender.

June was playing with Elliot on the living room floor, and when she saw me, she dropped her blocks and toddled into my lap. I wrapped her in my arms, and she let me cover her face with kisses.

"I'm so sorry, Peanut," I whispered into her damp ear, fresh tears spilling from my eyes. I pulled back from her and said, "Mommy should *not* throw plates. Don't let anyone treat you that way." My behavior made me feel like an abusive boyfriend, crawling back to her, promising I'd never do it again, even though we all knew I would.

The problem was, everyone kept telling me this was normal. I read motherhood memoirs and talked tentatively to other parents, who all praised me for apologizing and "making the repair." *Motherhood is really hard*, they said. *No one ever warns you how hard. You're doing a great job.* And I thought, *Okaaayyyy, but tell me* specifically *how you spend more than ten minutes with your kid without violently losing your mind?*

I knew babies cried, obviously I knew they cried, and I expected parenting to be hard, but if it were this hard for everyone, how come they could walk through town with happy babies gurgling in their strollers? If it were this hard for everyone, why did most families choose to have more than one kid? I already knew we wouldn't be doing this twice.

For the first two weeks of June's life, when she was quietly nestled in my arms, it was unfathomable to me that I would ever do anything to hurt her. She was perfect in every way and I loved her more than I could bear. I just didn't realize it was possible for her to hurt me too.

Her cries were knives in my eardrums and chest. Her touch on my body was fire. It was impossible to be the mother I imagined when her baby noises and baby demands made it feel like I had moved permanently inside the echoey, sticky nightmare of Chuck E. Cheese.

And I hated myself for even thinking that, which of course added another layer of guilt and shame. She was just being a baby, that's what babies do! But if I couldn't handle *this*, a normal baby with normal baby behaviors, then I'd already failed, before motherhood had even truly begun.

—15—

Normal

BY THIRTY-TWO I'D BEEN DIAGNOSED WITH ANXIETY, DEPRESSION, "high sensitivity," and "probably Tourette's," care of one psychiatrist who didn't seem to care much about the actual diagnosis because "There's no cure, so what does it matter?" As if the only reason to know yourself is so you can be fixed.

After I threw the plate, I knew I had to get back into therapy and I had to get back on meds, no matter the side effects. Over the years, I'd tried and gone off three different antidepressants— Wellbutrin, Prozac, and Lexapro—but even on the lowest possible doses, I experienced emotional numbness, racing heart, exacerbated tics, and a complete inability to sleep.

There was only one in-network psychiatrist's office near me, the Longshore Clinic, with a six-month wait list, so I DIYed my anger management while waiting for help. By now June was two, and life was less about surviving the hamster wheel of soothing, diaper changing, breastfeeding, and nap schedules and more about making it through day-to-day parenting. June's constant crying had decreased, and once a week we took her to the park or story time at the library or an indoor play space, but within fifteen minutes I was the weeping mess. The sun was too hot, the kids were too loud, my shoulder hurt from the heavy diaper bag, and while all the other parents gazed at their babies and clapped in time to "You Are My Sunshine," I was doing everything I could not to cover my ears and scream.

One afternoon, in one of my periods of hyperfixation on parenting theory, I stumbled across a podcast episode called "Psycho Mom." June and I were taking our morning walk around the neighborhood, and it was one of those days that made me worship at the altar of Northern California. The morning sun was turning each house into a buttery ball of gold. Every garden we passed smelled like jasmine.

"I think we all have a little experience with Psycho Mom," the host, Jamie Glowacki, was saying. "You're going about your parenting life and you are loving and gentle and you are trying not to yell and you are being all the things you think you're supposed to be— present and mindful and super conscious, and then your kid does that one thing *one more time*. And holy shit, the seventh gate of hell opens up and out comes Psycho Mom."

I stopped midstride outside my neighbor's house, the one with the blueberries I usually had to sprint past so June wouldn't yank them out by the handful.

"Psycho Mom yells. She may stomp, she may throw things across the room. She's catastrophic."

This is . . . normal?

"You guys, if Psycho Mom makes a semiregular appearance in your house, it's because you aren't letting out your feelings. You are building up steam." Jamie's advice was to find healthier ways to get rid of that pent-up energy, rather than letting it all out at once. She said we were allowed to set firm boundaries and show frustration when those boundaries are crossed. The rage happens when we put on our fake gentle-parent voice and pretend we're not mad. This leads to passive-aggressive behavior, which leads to "Psycho Mom."

"Do we really want to model stuffing our feelings?" she challenged.

No, I do not.

Jamie's advice made perfect sense.

That night, armed with my new knowledge, I started June's bedtime routine, committed to setting clear boundaries the moment I felt a twinge of irritation. Her room was a cozy cave, with birch trees Elliot had bought on Etsy and wedged into a corner, then wrapped in twinkly copper lights. June and I sat on the overstuffed rocking chair, tucked into this enchanted forest. She nursed for a few minutes, her pudgy hand resting on the swell of my chest. I admired her rubber band wrists and listened to her piglet grunts and swallows. This, I could always do.

When she finished, I opened our well-loved copy of *Goodnight Moon*, a board book that fit into the palm of my hand, its spine cracked and corners worn thin, exposing an underbelly of dusty brown cardboard.

"In the great green room . . ."

"What's that?" Her damp, chubby finger pointed at the thick page. I clutched the book tighter and bit the inside of my cheek. I hate being interrupted. Whether I'm focusing on work or watching a show or giving a monologue about my vegetable garden, an interruption feels like I've been happily gliding across a frozen lake when all at once the ice cracks and I'm plunged into the frigid water.

"Oh, that? That's a dollhouse so the little bunny can play." I steadied myself and kept reading. *"There was a telephone and . . ."*

A sucking sound as June pulled her thumb from her mouth. "What's that?"

My answer came out sharp and fast, quick as a paper cut. "That's a red balloon. I was getting to that. *There was a telephone and a . . ."*

"I want balloon!"

My heart leaped, a full jump into my throat before settling back somewhere near my collarbone. Was this the sign that Psycho Mom was coming? I'd *just* started reading.

"Yup," I said, trying to keep my voice maternal. "Balloons are great." *Set the boundary, Marian.* "No more questions, June, let me finish the book."

"Okay." Thumb popped back into her mouth.

"*There was a telephone and a red balloon, and a picture of . . . a cow! Jumping over the moon.*" My shoulders dropped a millimeter as I completed two full sentences, but I'd done this every night for the past year; I knew what was coming. It was like waiting for a fire alarm to beep, my body bracing for the sound, arrhythmic and inevitable.

Is *this* the rage trigger? Do I leave *now*? What am I supposed to do, just not do bedtime? Put her in her crib without a book? She'll scream! Do I make Elliot do it? But I feel like this *every* night and Elliot *just* did her bath and now he's cleaning the kitchen like a perfect angel husband. It's not fair to put more on him because I can't handle ten minutes alone with my kid. I just have to get through this book and then I can go to bed.

"*And three little bears—*"

"Bears!" she shouted. "Three bears!"

The rage the anger the fury the wild delirium whooshed up my body, cannonballed through my veins, down my arms, into my fingertips, and I flung the book across the room where it smashed into the wall.

We stared at the tattered cover splayed on the floor.

Elliot cracked open the door, but I was too mortified to register his expression. I kept my eyes down, studying the gray-and-white-striped sleep sack around June's shoulder.

"You okay?" he asked.

"No."

"Do you need me to finish?"

"Yes."

And he did. He always did. He took over and I fled, burrowing myself into bed once again.

Later that week, I mentioned this incident to my new therapist, Theresa.

"I'm trying to catch the rage before it starts, but it's *always* there. I can't read to June for more than sixty seconds before I'm throwing her book across the room and shoving her into Elliot's arms. I can't do the bare minimum of parenting." I hid my face in my palms.

"You know, you're allowed to tell June to not ask you questions while you read," Theresa said.

"I tried!" I wailed. "But she's a toddler! Toddlers ask questions! Isn't it my job to teach her?"

"Sure, but bedtime isn't the place for that. You can teach her that interrupting people isn't polite and to keep her questions until the end."

I liked this advice. That afternoon, I was filled with hope again. I just needed to set better boundaries!

Of course, the problem wasn't really that June asked too many questions or that I wasn't listening to my "triggers." The problem was that the underlying reason for the rage was hidden away and no one could tell me what it was.

SIX MONTHS LATER I got a call from the Longshore Clinic. One of their psychiatrists had an opening; would I like it? Yes, yes please god yes. I would do anything to become the mother June deserved. I would take any drug, endure any side effect.

That September I crawled into the office of Noelle Anderson, a pretty blonde in her forties whose office looked like a Florida beach condo. I told her about the years of erratic mood swings, my inability to keep a job, the revolving door of friendships, and, now that I had everything I wanted despite it all, a wanton rage toward my beautiful family. I walked her through my history on antidepressants and told her how Wellbutrin made my tics worse.

"Tics?" she asked.

"Oh, I've had them my whole life," I said, waving them off. "Usually eye blinking and nostril flaring. Sometimes I cycle through new ones, like locking my knees when I walk or drawing my shoulder blades together or rolling my neck. My last psychiatrist said it was likely a form of Tourette's but since there's no cure she didn't see the need to diagnose me."

"How do the tics feel, right before you do them?" She sat across from me in a small beige chair and started typing on the laptop perched on her knees.

"Like an itch. If I don't scratch, it gets bigger and bigger. It's like my eyes need air so I open them really wide and then blink hard."

"Do you do them consciously or unconsciously?"

"What do you mean?"

"For example, do you find yourself ticcing without realizing? Can you control them?"

"I always know I'm doing them. They're definitely conscious." Talking about blinking made my eyeballs itch. I kept them open a normal width and focused on Dr. Anderson, blinking at a normal rate. It's funny, writing this now, realizing how hard I was trying to look and act like a real girl as I verbally admitted to feeling anything but. "I can control them. I try not to tic around people, so I'll hold them in until someone's not looking at me or I'm alone. It just feels stressful to do it that way, like holding in a sneeze. I guess I find them comforting."

"Okay"—she clacked away at her keyboard—"I don't think your tics are Tourette's. Tourette's is uncontrollable and mostly involuntary. What you're describing sounds more like obsessive-compulsive disorder."

"OCD?" My skin tightened. Another diagnosis I didn't know what to do with. "That's a new one."

"Common OCD tics include compulsively washing your hands or turning the light switch on and off a specific number of times—"

"I definitely don't do that."

"Right, but it can also be like what you're describing." She peered at me over the top of her screen. "The desire to lock your knees at the beginning of a walk or to blink rapidly while watching a scary scene in a movie sounds more like compulsions than involuntary tics, and they can get worse with stress. Like being a new mom, for example." She gave me a small smile, I suppose to show me that she'd been there too, then turned back to her laptop. "I think you should try Lexapro again. You mentioned trying it a few years ago, so I'll start you on a lower dose. It can help the anxiety and depression, but it's also been used off-label to treat OCD, so you might see some relief. Wellbutrin isn't an SSRI, so I'm not surprised it made your tics worse."

I agreed to try the Lexapro again, and much to my surprise, it did what we wanted it to do. It helped my mood, which she called "episodic irritable depression, usually triggered by external stressors," almost overnight. I had more good days and more energy, but the kind of energy you get after drinking too much coffee. I was jumpy and twitching almost constantly, trying to shake the jitters out of my skin.

At my next appointment with Dr. Anderson, I explained that I found the medication helpful and didn't want to go off it, but I couldn't stand feeling so blown apart. She prescribed gabapentin, a nerve blocker that often works as an antianxiety med and might keep me from twitching.

My tics stayed the same, but the gabapentin made me so drowsy I'd fall asleep shortly after taking it, regardless of the time of day—which honestly wasn't the worst thing because of my brand-new insomnia. I passed entire nights staring at the ceiling, twitching and fidgeting, thoughts scattering like shards of glass. I dreaded climbing into bed, the only thing I had ever consistently looked forward to.

The next month she said, "Why don't we keep you on the gabapentin and have you take it at night? That should solve the sleep problem."

So I took a very low dose at night, so low that Dr. Anderson was surprised I noticed any side effects (my Lexapro was extremely low too; I never got above her lowest trial dosage). I was groggy in the morning, but at least I could keep both my Lexapro and the slightly improved mood that came with it.

But Lexapro can't perform miracles. I still screamed or got frustrated enough to throw something once a week. For a while, I told Dr. Anderson I was still struggling, but once we figured out a med cocktail that kept me level, she had only one recommendation left: self-care. *Are you exercising? Are you taking time for yourself? Have you tried yoga? Walk outside. Take a deep breath when you start feeling stressed.*

In our appointment summary notes she wrote, *Reviewed coping skills—eating regular meals, sleep hygiene, routine exercise, minimal alcohol intake, contact with friends and family.*

I didn't drink, my family was across the country, and I didn't have any friends. We'd run out of options, so I assumed this was just how it was going to be forever.

Instead of questioning Dr. Anderson or her advice, I judged myself. I must not be exercising *enough*. I'm not taking the right *kinds* of deep breaths. If only I had more friends, I wouldn't be so stressed.

Self-care felt ludicrous, like putting a Band-Aid on a severed limb. In therapy with Theresa, I struggled to articulate the battle in my brain.

"But *the sound*. How am I supposed to take deep breaths when the sound of June's crying claws itself into my skin?"

"I know, the sound of a baby crying is terrible," said Theresa. "It's designed to make us sit up and pay attention. It's perfectly normal to feel dysregulated."

But you don't understand! I screamed inside. *It's not terrible. It's* unbearable. *I literally cannot stand to hear it. It feels like death, like being sucked into space, like I've been strapped into that torture device from* The Princess Bride.

Still, I was told: This is normal. Yes, of course, parenting is hard.

Everyone hates the sound of a baby crying. All moms feel rage. Welcome to motherhood.

I READ A STORY recently about a woman named Ashley. After her first baby was born, Ashley had severe postpartum depression, anxiety, and OCD. At one point, things got so bad she had to be hospitalized. Her doctors explained how serious things were, but her friends all said some variation of "Oh well, motherhood is so hard, who wouldn't feel terrible? It's so anxiety-provoking to have children!"

"It really made me question myself," Ashley said. "Like, is everyone actually in this boat? Am I weak, am I not cut out to be a mother if this feels out of control? If we're all in the same boat, why am I such a whiner? Should I just be toughing it out—because maybe everyone is as despairing and incapacitated as I am, who knows, I'm not in their head?"

This normalization of women's stress and pain has created one of the biggest barriers to diagnosis—not just for autism, for *anything*.

In the incredible, must-read book *Doing Harm*, author Maya Dusenbery writes about how the widespread myth that menstrual pain is normal has drastically delayed the diagnosis of endometriosis, a painful disease where tissue grows outside the uterus. Teenagers with severe menstrual cramps are told that they simply haven't learned how to handle a normal period. "Yet studies suggest," Maya writes, "that about 70 percent of teens who complain of [painful periods] are eventually diagnosed with endometriosis."

Which was exactly my own experience.

The pain started in high school. When I was fifteen, I fell to my bedroom floor one evening after a sudden, sharp stab on the right side of my pelvis. Mom rushed me to the emergency room, where an old man jabbed inside me with such force that I lay there weeping on the exam table.

"Ovarian cysts," he said, and sent me home.

This wasn't a complete surprise. Every woman on my mother's side has endometriosis. Mom had an ovary removed, and my aunt and cousin had hysterectomies, so it made sense that my reproductive system was already turning on me. That year, my gynecologist put me on the birth control pill and sent me on my way.

Even so, the pain got worse in college. I saw an ob-gyn off campus, but she said I was too young to have endometriosis. I explained that every woman in my family had it, my periods were debilitating, I couldn't have sex without crying, and I'd had a cyst rupture in high school, but none of it mattered. She shook her head and said it wasn't possible. I was "too young" and I likely had an STD. Without even waiting for the swab results, she prescribed doxycycline to treat my "obvious chlamydia." A few days later, the test came back negative, because of course it did, but it still couldn't possibly be endometriosis, she said. "You should see a gastroenterologist for a colonoscopy."

Only after testing negative for Crohn's disease could I convince her to perform the laparoscopic surgery that would diagnose and remove the endometriosis. When I woke up from surgery, she announced, "I found scar tissue on your fallopian tubes and the wall of your abdomen." As if she were telling me something I didn't already know.

Relieved to have a diagnosis, I smiled. Until I discovered that she didn't remove said scar tissue, just stitched me back up and suggested a drug called Lupron that would force me through a temporary menopause. I was twenty.

I declined the Lupron and muscled through five years of "treatment": birth control pills that skipped my period and would theoretically slow the growth of the endometrial tissue, fistfuls of ibuprofen, and scalding hot water bottles. When I was twenty-five, I tried again with a different doctor in a different hospital in a different state and was horrified to be put through the entire diagnostic process again, despite imagery from the first surgery that *proved I had endometriosis*.

Before my new doctor would even consider "looking for endometriosis," she made me take a weekend pain management class that involved stretching and deep breathing. When that didn't magically fix ten years of pain, she instructed me to track my liquid intake and urine output for three days. I measured everything I drank and peed into a disposable measuring cup to make sure nothing was wrong with my kidneys. When *those* results came back negative, she did a casual but painful session of vaginal physical therapy that involved a large wand and a machine that beeped.

"You need to relax," she said, prodding inside me. I gritted my teeth and tried not to cry.

Only after months chasing peripheral diagnoses did she agree to the laparoscopic surgery and—this is key—*the actual removal of the scar tissue that was causing my pain*. To her credit, she did a beautiful job, but did it really need to take ten years, three time-consuming tests, countless medications, a weekend class, four incorrect diagnoses, and two surgeries to take my first suggestion seriously?

If it sounds like I'm angry, it's because I am. But at least my life wasn't at risk. At least I kept all my organs and bones and limbs.

In August 2018, my friend Dana woke up and noticed that her right arm was tingling. When the sensation didn't go away after a couple of days, she called her doctor and made the first available appointment, two weeks out.

The next morning, Dana couldn't lift her arm above her head. Her fingernails had turned blue. Terrified, Dana's husband rushed her to urgent care. The attending doctor, a man in his fifties, didn't seem concerned.

"Dana's dad had a heart attack and died from an aortic aneurysm," Dana's husband pressed. "How do we know this isn't cardiac related?"

The doctor looked at Dana with a sarcastic grin and replied, "Because you'd be dead."

Dana started crying.

"Oh, honey," said the doctor. "You seem anxious. Do you have anxiety?"

Dana nodded.

"That's all this is: anxiety and a pinched nerve from bad posture. After a few personal training sessions, you'll see."

Embarrassed, Dana tried to ignore the tingling in her arm as she researched personal trainers. Five days passed. The swelling and discoloration were now so pronounced, people noticed just by glancing at her. Dana could barely feel her hand. She called her primary care doctor and asked if there was any way they could fit her in their schedule early. The doctor was booked, they said, but the physician's assistant could see her.

The physician's assistant took one look at Dana and called an ambulance. Dana arrived at the emergency room, where a team of surgeons came in to examine her. They spoke in hushed tones, but she knew what they were talking about—amputation. They agreed to wait until the results of her ultrasound.

The ultrasound revealed that Dana had several large blood clots in her shoulder and arm. The most likely cause was thoracic outlet syndrome—a compression of her subclavian vein by her first rib. If the first urgent care doctor hadn't dismissed Dana and instead had sent her straight to the emergency room, they would likely have been able to use a "clot buster"—an IV injection that could break up the clots inside her veins—but it was too late. She needed surgery to remove part of her rib. Luckily, none of the clots had broken off and traveled, which could have been fatal.

The recovery from her rib resection was excruciating and came with a side of neuralgia, a constant burning sensation in her side due to nerve damage from the surgery. For ninety days she was on blood thinners—any bump, cut, or nosebleed could have sent her back to the hospital—but thankfully, she was going to be okay.

After her recovery, Dana consulted with a malpractice lawyer who told her that yes, the situation was scary and unfortunate, but she didn't have a case. If her arm had been amputated, or if she'd had a pulmonary embolism and died, then the urgent care doctor could be held accountable. "As far as I know," Dana told me, "he's still practicing and could still be belittling and dismissing women today."

It's a tale as old as time. For centuries, women's unexplained symptoms fell under the catchall diagnosis *hysteria*, and while that particular term has fallen out of fashion, it's been replaced with euphemisms like *anxiety* and *stress*. Sometimes symptoms are blamed on our delicate lady problems like menstrual cramps, menopause, or new motherhood. "Sometimes, other aspects of their identity seem to take center stage," writes Maya Dusenbery. "Fat women report that any ailment is blamed on their weight; trans women find that all their symptoms are attributed to hormone therapy; black women are stereotyped as addicts looking for prescription drugs, their reports of pain doubted entirely."

Psychotherapist Rebecca Jay knows this all too well. When Rebecca was seventeen, they contracted bronchitis and walking pneumonia. When their cough didn't go away, doctors shrugged and told them, "If you lost weight, you wouldn't have this many coughing fits." For five years Rebecca suffered, endlessly going to doctors, looking for relief. They were diagnosed with bronchospasms, gastroesophageal reflux disease, asthma, and "a touch of pneumonia." Every time they asked questions, the treatment was the same. "My doctor felt that losing weight would help," Rebecca wrote in 2015. "Maybe I could try yoga, or swimming. It was very hard to continue to move when you can barely breathe."

Even though Rebecca had started coughing blood, the doctors' dismissals came so fast and fierce that Rebecca started thinking they were a hypochondriac and began researching inpatient facilities for mental health.

Then one day Rebecca landed in the emergency room with a fever. After a CT scan and an X-ray, the doctors found a tumor in their bronchial tube. Rebecca had cancer. Two weeks later Rebecca had surgery to remove their lung, "the bottom half of which was a black, rotting piece of dead tissue."

"When my surgeon told me a diagnosis five years prior could've saved my lung, I remember a feeling of complete and utter rage. Because I remembered the five years I spent looking for some kind of reason why I was always coughing, always sick. Most of all, I remembered being consistently told that the reason I was sick was because I was fat."

Regardless of which external attribute is to blame, the through line in our experiences is identical: we can't be trusted to know when something is wrong with our bodies.

The research tells this same exhausting story. Women are diagnosed *years* later than men with over seven hundred diseases. We die at higher rates from heart attacks, which are still somehow seen as primarily happening to men, despite coronary disease being the leading cause of death in women. When men have chronic pain, they're described as brave and stoic, while women are emotional and hysterical. Many drugs were never even tested on women, making us more likely to experience adverse reactions to medications. Even lab rats are overwhelmingly male because apparently, female hormones "mess with the data." As if over half the population is some sort of special case.

So it shouldn't come as a surprise that this gender bias bleeds into the world of developmental disorders. In the same way our physical pain is brushed off as "the anxiety of being a woman," so are our reports of sensory overload, social confusion, repetitive behaviors, and inflexibility. The result? Eighty percent of autistic girls remain undiagnosed by the time they're eighteen.

The fact that I found out at all is a miracle.

—16—

The Keys

ONE YEAR BEFORE MY DIAGNOSIS, I SAW COMEDIAN HANNAH GADSBY live in San Francisco. They were touring their new show, *Douglas*, in which they revealed they were autistic. I was sitting in the audience, tucked into a worn red theater seat, just right of center stage at the Palace of Fine Arts. My cheeks hurt from laughing so hard.

"To give you an idea of what it feels like to be on the spectrum," Hannah was saying, "it feels like being the only sober person in a room full of drunks. Or the other way around. Basically, everyone is operating on a wavelength you can't quite key into." On the screen behind them, where they'd been giving a casual art history lecture, Hannah projected an image of Giotto's *The Meeting at the Golden Gate*, in which an old woman in a black shroud stands scowling in the background of a festive scene. "To give you a visual? This woman." The audience erupted into laughter.

"Honestly, the day I was formally diagnosed with autism was a very good day. Because it felt like I'd been handed the keys to the city of me . . . Why I felt such a profound sense of isolation my entire life, despite trying so hard to be part of the team. And that is a big thing about being on the spectrum. It is lonely. I find it very difficult to connect to others, because my brain takes me to places where nobody else lives."

If this were a movie, you might imagine me sitting in the dark of the theater. The spotlight would shift from Hannah to me, and the light would get progressively brighter until an expression of pure bliss and relief flooded my face as you watched the moment I recognized that *I* was autistic too.

Alas, in the real world, I didn't so much as flinch.

Hannah handed me the keys to my own city, and I looked down at them shining in my hand, then looked back up, blank faced and confused.

It wasn't only their words that should have sent me down a spiral of self-discovery, but their actions. Early in the show, a woman in the audience yelled toward the stage, "I love you, Hannah!"

Hannah was midsentence, and I watched the interruption plunge them through that frozen lake of icy water. I watched their brain glitch, then switch from the practiced, comforting rhythm of their performance to the sensory experience of every person in that auditorium—our sniffles and shifts and crinkling candy wrappers. A thousand wet eyeballs glued onto them.

Hannah's expression slackened. They tried to keep going but tripped over their next words. Then they grimaced. Tripped again. This all happened in a matter of seconds, but it was as if I were watching myself on that stage, reading a book to June before flinging it across the room.

After a minute of fumbling, Hannah stopped.

"Please don't do that," they said out into the dark toward the voice of the faceless fan. "Even to say something nice. It makes me lose my place. I can't perform if I hear you yelling."

I'd never seen anyone, never mind a public figure, stumble so visibly after auditory stimulation. In fact, I'd always seen the opposite: sitcom moms gossiping on the phone with their besties while three sticky children bang on pots in the background, without so much as a flinch.

Tense silence rippled through the auditorium and Hannah's next few sentences were stilted, but two minutes later it was as if nothing had happened. We laughed so hard we cried. I doubt anyone else in the audience remembers that moment.

But I remember. And even if I hadn't yet drawn the connection between the word *autism* and myself, I had just watched someone's brain react to the world the way mine always had. They didn't apologize for it either. I watched them ask for what they needed and get it without much fanfare. To my surprise, people didn't flee screaming from the auditorium because Hannah Gadsby set a boundary.

I wish I'd driven home that night and googled, "Am I autistic?" but it would be another year before that phrase graced my search history (alongside "How to get a toddler to eat vegetables" and "Leather jackets without zippers on the sleeves"). Instead, the connection filed itself away in my brain, waiting for the day someone wouldn't just hand me the keys but unlock the door and kick it wide open.

IT WAS JULY AND I was thirty-four, sitting at my kitchen table waiting for the kettle to boil. I had one ear out for the quiet pause that signaled that the water was about to start bubbling, phone in my hand, scrolling through nothing, looking for entertainment to occupy my brain in the few open minutes between work and a fresh cup of tea. We'd recently left San Francisco for Portland, Oregon. June was in preschool and I had somehow lasted at a full-time job for four whole years after lucking my way into a virtual company. My life, despite it all, had fallen into a comforting rhythm.

My thumb paused over a video my friend Delia had posted to Instagram. In the video, Delia's frozen frame showed her dark-blond hair in a braid over her right shoulder. She was wearing a gray tank with a sports bra underneath. I usually hate watching videos people make for social media—I usually scroll by quickly, unable to meet even digital eyes. But not that afternoon, not in the space of time it took to boil water for tea. I let the video play and tapped the speaker icon.

"So." She exhaled sharply with a laugh, uncomfortable and nervous. "I have been . . . diagnosed with autism." A little half smile, then she glanced away, out a window, evidenced by the light on her skin. "Life is so weird."

The palm gripping my phone became damp. My body hunched closer, my nose practically touching the screen. I turned up the volume. I heard the water in the kettle start moving faster. Delia was still talking. She'd had struggles her whole life, she was saying, so many struggles people didn't know about, and what she knows now is that what she was doing was called masking, trying to imitate other people in order to survive.

The kettle was on a full boil. I usually got up before it clicked off, the anticipation before the click always making me restless because I could never predict exactly when it would happen, but this time I barely registered the noise. Delia's voice was shooting down dormant wires in my brain, sending sparks in different directions, illuminating dark and forgotten spaces. My brain lit up like a Christmas tree. Like a baseball stadium. Like those images of Earth from space.

"It feels good to finally have some answers about myself," she said. "I encourage anyone to seek answers. I feel relieved. I burst into tears when the psychologist told me. Thank god for my son Mateo. If it weren't for him getting diagnosed, I probably would have never known. I probably would have struggled a lot more. It would have been a longer, harder road. He saved my life."

A man's voice called from the background, then the video turned off, the screen went gray, and Instagram asked if I wanted to watch it again.

I pushed myself up from the table, which rocked underneath me. I walked to the kettle. Grabbed my favorite mug, the blue-gray one with the thick handle. I dropped in a tea bag. Poured water over the top. The steam bloomed around me, and while the tea steeped, I stared at the knives lined in a crooked row on the wall. It looked like my house, but I was suddenly a stranger in it.

Elliot's footsteps thumped down the stairs. He rounded into the kitchen and tapped my hip as he passed before grabbing a granola bar from the pantry. I didn't move.

"You okay?" he asked. I knew his eyes were on me and I saw the tilt of his head out of my side vision.

A noise exited the back of my throat. My intention was for it to sound like *mm-hmm* but it came out strangled, like the embarrassing moan you make when you're drifting into sleep. The eventual weeks of research, the doctors, the online tests, even the official diagnosis that would come were all arbitrary.

I knew.

I finally knew exactly who I was.

FOR A WEEK, I didn't say anything to anyone, not even Elliot. I kept the news hidden inside myself, tucked up like a delicate sprout, terrified the lightest rain, the gentlest puff of wind would stunt its growth, causing it to wither and die before it ever grew past its cotyledons.

Outside, Portland cooked. It was 120 degrees in our backyard. The hydrangeas wilted, then crisped. The blueberries shriveled on their branches. The news told us to close the windows and curtains, stay hydrated, leave water out for the birds and bees and people without shelter. The view from our back picture window looked like a perfect summer day, but moving from the house to the car was like crawling into an oven and pulling the door shut behind you.

That week, I sat on the phone with my boss, listening to her brainstorm new marketing strategies, and I felt a creeping, unfamiliar contempt. She cracked a joke and I didn't laugh. She assigned a project I usually would have loved and I just grunted that I'd handle it.

I don't belong here! I wanted to scream. *You and I are not the same!* I pressed my lips together until my teeth left indents inside my mouth.

At night I ran through moments from my past. Lining up my glass animals in neat rows organized by species and size, dusting them every night in my childhood bedroom. Hiding in corners, hiding in tents, behind the couch, away from people and activities that were supposed to be fun. Reading a book and feeling the urge to repeat certain words out loud—the ones I suspected would feel good coming out of my throat and into the air where I could hear their shapes in my ears. Wombat. Crystal. Edge.

Every tiny moment swooped in, battering me down, drowning me in swells of long-forgotten memories.

And then, once the storm was over, once this new knowledge had infiltrated my veins and rewired my brain, I started to read.

THE FIRST THING I did, of course, was turn to Google.

"Am I autistic?" I asked.

"Take this free autism test and get instant results," Google said.

I took a dozen tests, right-clicking each one until my browser window was too full to see their titles. Each was a version of the Autism Spectrum Quotient, a self-administered and slightly outdated questionnaire used to measure autistic traits in adults without intellectual disabilities. Most of the tests included a number of statements that I answered on a scale from "Definitely Agree" to "Definitely Disagree."

> I prefer to do things with others rather than on my own.
> Other people frequently tell me that what I've said is impolite, even though I think it is polite.

I frequently get so strongly absorbed in one thing that I
    lose sight of other things.
I often notice small sounds when others do not.
I find it hard to make new friends.

Again and again the tests tabulated their results and I bounced
my knees as the page loaded.

"Significant autistic traits," they told me.

How could this be? How could I, at thirty-four years old, just . . .
not know? Autistic people were eight-year-old boys who didn't talk,
or who did talk but only about trains or robots or dinosaurs. Autistic
people screamed in public and flapped their hands and banged their
heads against the wall. My face flooded with shame at the thought.
I was a monster.

*Oh boo hoo, you find conversation awkward and eye contact hard.
How sad for you.*

*You don't have any friends because you're selfish and mean, not because
there's anything clinically different about you.*

I worried that I was trying to align myself with the oppressed to
feel special and excuse a lifetime of shitty behavior.

But.

Hannah.

Delia.

And they weren't the only ones. During the last few years, I'd
become obsessed with autistic creators on TV and social media, including Josh Thomas, an Australian writer and comedian, whose
show *Everything's Gonna Be Okay* is about a character version of his
real-life persona discovering he's autistic late in life. Josh was charming and creative and quirky and relatable, and I had been devouring
everything he had ever created.

Because of course I have.

I kept thinking about that song "Escape (The Piña Colada
Song)," which tells the story of a couple who each secretly purchase

separate personal ads in the newspaper only to discover they'd been falling back in love with each other the whole time. That's how I felt, realizing I'd been drawn toward this community not by chance or curiosity—but because *I already belonged to them*.

Day after day, I watched videos and read stories of late-diagnosed women. I scanned message boards for glimpses of myself. I learned that almost everything we know about autism is based on straight white boys. In 1943, Dr. Leo Kanner did the first study on autistic children, whom he categorized as having a "powerful desire for aloneness and sameness." Only three of the eleven children in the study were girls. The next year, a psychiatrist in Vienna named Hans Asperger started researching the idea of autism as a spectrum, identifying a segment of autistic kids who acted like "little professors" and whose intense absorption could provide valuable contributions to our society. None of the children in his initial study were girls.

In the decades that followed, we've remained obsessed with the idea that autism occurs only in boys and the rare girl whose symptoms must be "severe" enough to qualify. As recently as 2002, British psychologist Simon Baron-Cohen proposed that autism was the result of an "extreme male brain." According to him, male brains are better at systems and pattern-spotting, whereas female brains are better at feelings and empathy, so if you're autistic you must have a REALLY REALLY SUPER MANLY brain.

Stereotypes sprang up in a line of zealous actors gagging for their Oscar. In *Rain Man*, Dustin Hoffman gave us the first on-screen depiction of autism; his character, Raymond, could magically count hundreds of toothpicks as they fell to the floor. Sheldon Cooper from *The Big Bang Theory* is considered autistic-coded. He's rude and condescending with little empathy for others, and he has difficulty socializing and a strong preference for routine. He's even obsessed with trains. But it's all okay because he's brilliant! Then there's Elon Musk, Certified Real Man™, who came out publicly in 2021 as "having Asperger's" during the most painful SNL monologue I've ever seen, further reinforcing the image of autism as an awkward but genius white guy in tech (unless he's a high-needs but genius white guy in an institution, of course).

Do these stereotypes stem from the fact that autism really is a predominantly male condition, or is autism considered a predominantly male condition thanks to these stereotypes? Most experts agree that autism is genetic; while we still don't really know what causes it, some studies have suggested it takes a bigger genetic "hit" for girls to show the more classic autism symptoms than it does for boys.

I spoke with Dr. Maria Kontaridis, currently the executive director at Masonic Medical Research Institute in New York and an associate professor of medicine at Harvard Medical School. She explained that many of the genes that cause autism are found on the X chromosome; since women have two, one can mask the other and compensate for the mutation. I've sometimes heard this called the "female protective effect."

But it's also not that simple. "The truth is, we still don't know so much," Maria told me. "What I can tell you is that there are numerous cases where the 'highly functioning' form of autism is passed from father to son, which means it cannot simply be X-linked. As such, females and males are equally likely to have an Autism Level 1 disorder, what used to be known as Asperger's."

She also reminded me that historically, research has looked only at male samples, including male mice and rats. "We would just extrapolate and assume women behaved the same way, and we now know that's not true. We overlooked 50 percent of the demographic."

As awareness of "female autism" has become slightly more mainstream and diagnosis criteria slightly less biased, the rate of diagnosed girls has inched ever higher. In 2012, boys were 4.7 times more likely to be diagnosed autistic than girls. In just over a decade, that number has dropped to 3.8. In a 2020 analysis of over 226,000 eight-year-olds, the number of autistic girls was the highest ever recorded.

I learned it wasn't only girls who were being missed, but autistic people from all marginalized communities. Gay, nonbinary, and trans people are less likely to be diagnosed. Black, Brown, and Indigenous kids are less likely to be diagnosed. And while some label this group of late-diagnosed autistics as having the "female autism phenotype," which is essentially a list of "milder," more socially acceptable symptoms, I prefer Devon Price's language of "masked Autism," which he defines as "a camouflaged version of the disorder that's still widely neglected by researchers, mental health providers, and Autism organizations that aren't led by Autistic people."

"When I use the term masked Autism," Devon writes, "I'm referring to any presentation of the disability that deviates from the standard image we see in most diagnostic tools and nearly all media portrayals of Autism. Since Autism is a pretty complex and multifaced disorder, that covers a lot of different traits, which can manifest in many different ways."

I learned that autistic girls are a group most likely to mask, simply by nature of the way we're raised. From birth we're enrolled in an intensive, lifelong training of putting others first. Sit still. Be quiet. Be helpful. Be agreeable. Keep tidy. Be pretty. Be friendly, but not *too* friendly—that's flirting, don't be a slut. We can't walk down the street without strangers ordering us to smile. So on top of suppressing any unladylike behaviors, autistic girls double down on the mask by suppressing our stims, our sensory needs, our interests. We force eye contact and conversation and grit our teeth through the noise and the light and the itchy tags and sock seams and underwires digging into our rib cages. Because why the hell not? We're shoving it all down anyway. What's a little eye twitching when you're already caked in layers of makeup, Spanx, and exhaustion?

While autistic boys mask too, the socialization of girls makes us particularly vulnerable. "Boys will be boys" was the unspoken (and sometimes spoken) motto of my childhood, with no equivalent catchphrase to explain my behavior. If I begged for quiet in the family minivan, I was aggressive, but my brothers yelling over each other about bombs were not.

I learned autistic girls are more likely to wear masks because all girls are forced to wear them, from the moment we open our eyes. The only difference is what the mask is hiding.

SINCE THAT AFTERNOON IN Mr. Bacon's classroom closet, I'd never fully trusted my own interpretation of myself. I was always surprised when someone accused me of being rude, selfish, or moody. It wasn't that I didn't believe them: I *only* believed them. I believed them to the point of dismissing my own instincts. Clearly, my self view was flawed, and the question of my autism wasn't any different.

Despite the gut feeling that washed over me while watching Delia's video, and the confirmation from dozens of self-tests, I still wanted an outside expert to see all of me and articulate exactly why I showed up in the world so differently from everyone else. I needed to know for sure, and I didn't trust my ability to interpret each convoluted symptom through the lens of my own experiences. So back to Google I went. "Adult autism diagnosis in Portland, Oregon."

I called and emailed every clinic I could find.

"Sorry, our wait list is at least eighteen months—we're not even adding new patients to it."

"Thanks for contacting me. I'm not assessing adults at this time."

One clinic seemed shocked I was even asking.

"You want an *adult* assessment?"

"Yes."

"For your adult child?"

"No, for myself."

"Oh no. No no no, we don't do that." She practically hung up on me.

I had no idea where else to go. I now believe that self-diagnosis is perfectly valid, and the path to an official medical diagnosis is littered with unnecessary expense and trauma for marginalized communities, but at that point in my early understanding of autism, all I wanted was someone to watch me as I carried out my day, to take a look inside my brain and tell me one way or the other why I'd felt like an alien my whole life. If this pattern sounds familiar, it's because hello, welcome to this whole book.

I decided to bring the question to Dr. Anderson, whom I was now seeing via telehealth.

A few minutes before our monthly check-in, I opened our Zoom link and sat at my laptop staring at my own face, waiting for Dr. Anderson to log on. My teeth chattered. I tightened my jaw, only for the shakes to travel into my arms and hands. I was vibrating out of my chair.

What the hell are you thinking? my brain berated me. *Autism?* Suddenly I was terrified of being "that patient," the one who thinks two weeks of research on WebMD somehow counteracts decades of medical experience.

Dr. Anderson appeared on-screen.

"Hey!" I said, way too chipper. "How are you?"

"Good. How have you been?"

"Fine, fine." I noticed that her home office had two French doors painted black, and I'd just painted all the doors in my hallway black, so I talked at her for five minutes about how much I liked her doors. She eventually cut me off to run through our usual appointment checklist: How's your anxiety? How are your tics? Your sleep? Your anger? Your exercise habits? Are you getting enough sleep?

I'd gone off Lexapro, and with the pandemic and our move to Oregon, she and I were ending our time together after nearly two years.

It was now or never.

Looking at her face looking at me made me not want to broach the subject, so I minimized Zoom and focused on my desktop: a generic mountainscape provided by Apple, littered with screenshots and half-written books and downloaded forms I couldn't remember whether I'd ever sent.

"Anything else?" she asked.

"Yeah—um. One thing." I swallowed. "What do you know about autism?" *Fuck.* I was chickening out, unable to be direct about what I really wanted to know.

"Hmm," she said. "Not a lot. That's not really my area. Why do you ask?"

I told her a choppy version of the story. My friend was diagnosed in her thirties; she and I were really similar.

"What specifically feels like autism to you?" Her tone was odd, the way you'd talk to a child. At least, I think it was. My mind sank into that familiar place of terror, where every word out of my mouth was a grenade. Would it land quietly in the grass or explode?

"Well . . ." God, why was this so hard? I felt like I was having to defend my thesis, not have an intelligent adult conversation with a doctor I'd known and liked for two years. "I get kind of awkward in groups? And then there are the tics?" I couldn't think of a single other autistic trait. I'd forgotten everything I'd researched.

"That sounds a lot like social anxiety, and as for your tics, I've said before that feels more in line with OCD."

"Yeah, okay." This was so embarrassing. I couldn't wait to get off the phone.

"Plus," she added, "you're married and have a child. You've always been charming with me. People with autism have a very hard time living a normal life."

We finished quickly after that. At 4:45, I shut my laptop and slipped on my sandals and drove the ten minutes to June's preschool to pick her up. The heat wave had subsided, but it was still too hot to stand outside for long, and June took forever to get into her car seat. I snapped at her to hurry so I could start the car and blast the air-conditioning directly into my face.

We ate dinner. Ran her bath. I read June a book and managed not to throw it across the room. I collapsed into bed and numbed out on *The Crown*. I rubbed my feet together until they were tingly and numb. I matched my breaths to Elliot's as we fell asleep. Dr. Anderson's words repeated in the back of my mind. *Charming with a family. Charming with a family.*

And then, much to my surprise, a whisper of something—a thought in my own voice overriding her all-knowing doctoral power, easing my rocking body into stillness.

I didn't believe her.

—17—

The Door

BY AUGUST, AFTER ALL MY REGULAR DOCTORS AND THERAPISTS HAD stared at me with blank, slightly worried expressions, and the first dozen pages of Google had turned up nothing but childhood learning centers, play therapists, and nonprofits, I turned to the people I should have asked in the first place—the women who had come before me.

I joined communities on Reddit and Facebook with names like "aspergirls" and "Autistic PDX," hoping they could point me toward someone who worked with adults. If I was having a hard time, others probably were too. I typed the word "diagnosed" into a Facebook group's search bar and up popped hundreds of threads: "Who diagnosed you?" "How do you know for sure that you're autistic?" "Can anyone tell me WHERE I can find someone to test me?" In the comments were link after link of doctors who not only worked with adults but specialized in "masked" autistics who'd learned how to hide themselves under layers of camouflage.

Jackpot.

I emailed three doctors whose names I read most frequently.

My name is Marian, I wrote, *and I found your name in a Facebook group for autistic women. I suspect I may be on the spectrum and am*

looking for a doctor to confirm or deny. Are you accepting new patients?
How does the assessment process work?

One doctor, Wendela Marsh, was based in Oregon. She'd written eight books on autism, married an autistic man, had two autistic kids, and spent decades assessing autistic children in California public schools. Reading her website made my shoulders drop from where they'd been hovering around my ears.

> *Do you wonder if you might be on the autism spectrum? Perhaps you've felt different your whole life and struggled with social communication, trying to fit in. Did it seem like everybody else had a secret rule book for how to make friends? If you are intelligent and pretty good at "masking" or pretending to be "normal," it's no surprise that you weren't diagnosed as a child. Now, we know a lot more about autism. It looks different for cisgender women, trans, and non-binary folk than it looks for cis men, different for adults than for children, and different for those with average or higher intelligence than for those with intellectual disability.*

If anyone could give me an answer, it would be Dr. Marsh.

She responded within a day. No, she didn't have a wait list, and yes, she could see me within the next few weeks. Why didn't we hop on a call for a short get-to-know-you chat so she could answer any questions?

On that first Zoom, Dr. Marsh's face filled my screen, and I immediately liked the look of her. She wore thick red-framed glasses and had short white hair with a bright blue streak in front. Something about her expression made me think she must take her grandkids on RV road trips every summer and have a little free library in her front yard. Even though we wouldn't be meeting in person, I felt comforted knowing she was forty-five minutes away.

I told her about Delia's Instagram video and my instant full-body reaction to the word *autism*. I told her about Dr. Anderson's dismissal and all the research I'd been doing since. Dr. Marsh explained that her assessment would include two Zoom observational interviews and five questionnaires designed to look for the core traits of autism, including social impairment, sensory processing patterns, and repetitive and restricted behaviors and interests. She'd be using a few standard diagnostic tests, plus three she wrote herself.

"You wrote the tests yourself?" I asked.

"Yes. Some of the official tests have questions that don't actually relate to the diagnostic criteria. They relate to people's ideas about what autism should look like. Asking a question like, 'Do you have good hygiene?' is not diagnostic, so I wrote a series of questionnaires that get to the answer in a different way, to get to the truth behind what's been going on. So if the diagnostic criteria is about social initiations and responsiveness, my question might be, 'When I try to flirt, it doesn't always land the way I intended,' or 'I can't tell if someone is trying to flirt with me or be friendly.'"

Then she added, "Most of the tests published for autism are for children, and many of the ones for adults are normed on a predominantly male population, which can miss women and other genders."

Often, when children are assessed for autism, assessors look for stereotyped behaviors, like flapping hands, when in reality, autistic behaviors can be as varied as the people themselves. "Instead of flapping her hands," Dr. Marsh explained, "a girl might be biting the inside of her cheek or curling her toes, but nobody can see that. Instead of trains, she might be obsessed with makeup." Those girls get missed. And missing them further stereotypes an autistic person as a boy who flaps his hands and can't stop talking about trains, when there are girls who flare their nostrils and can talk at you for thirty minutes about how Emma Bunton wasn't *actually* part of the original Spice Girls lineup, which was called "Touch" before they changed their name in 1995.

At the time, the cost of an assessment with Dr. Marsh was $2,000. I called my insurance to see if they would cover it.

"A *what* assessment?" the agent asked me over the crackly line.

"A-u-t-i-s-m."

"Ohhhhh, X-ray."

"AUTISM."

"My apologies. Yes, here it is. An X-ray. Your copay will be $20."

I hung up and fought the urge to fling my phone out the window just to hear it shatter the glass.

In the end, I got lucky. Not because insurance covered my assessment (it didn't, and most plans in the United States don't), but because I could afford an assessment without bankrupting my family. I was lucky to find someone at all who specialized in my particular flavor of neurodivergence, lucky to have a validating experience that didn't send me deeper into a hole of confusion and isolation.

After thinking it over for a week and wondering whether self-diagnosis would be enough, I put the assessment on my credit card and hoped to god this would bring me some peace.

I REMEMBER ONLY FLASHES from that first observational interview with Dr. Marsh. Laptop propped on the chair in front of me, my body curled under a blanket on the couch, feet tucked under me like a baby hedgehog. Dr. Marsh was kind and almost motherly, but I couldn't stop shaking. I'm still not sure why I was so nervous. Was I afraid that she'd judge me? Worried that I was blowing my differences way out of proportion? Or did I know, deep down, that I was on the brink of a new life? I felt perched on the edge of everything.

Until that day, I'd always tried to hide my true feelings so I could look capable, but here, with Dr. Marsh, I knew that in order for her to assess me correctly, I had to crack open a piece of myself and show her the dark and rotting insides.

The first hour of questions conjured memories I'd long forgotten. For instance, the "special interests" stereotype of autism had never quite felt relatable. I'd never had one singular passion that consumed my every conversation. Or so I thought. Until I remembered my collections—jars full of sea glass; the hundreds of wildlife fact-file cards I pored over every night when I was ten; the thick three-ring binder full of Leonardo DiCaprio photographs I'd printed off the internet when I was thirteen; the glass animals I dusted and rearranged daily, while letting weeks of laundry pile up in the corner. Then, as an adult, my obsessions with gardening, horseback riding, knitting, backyard chicken keeping, hot yoga, rock tumbling—each lasting six months to a year before I latched on to another interest with such fervor, I'd be an expert within the week.

When Dr. Marsh asked about my body awareness, a strong memory surfaced from my elementary and middle school years: I had frequent pee accidents in public places. Once, in third grade during reading circle. Another time, a few months before my friends dumped me in the closet, I'd peed all over the hardwood floor of Katie K.'s foyer. I remember the two of us sopping it up with bath towels, while the heat of my shame spread faster than we could wipe away. Another time, I was trick-or-treating with Chelsea, when I realized that if I didn't pee *right now* I was going to do it on the sidewalk. At the next house I begged the owner to use her bathroom. I didn't make it. I peed all over this strange woman's tile, stuffed my soaked tights into her garbage can, and fled, leaving a standing puddle on the floor. I was thirteen.

How had I forgotten this? How had I never considered the incision that had always existed between my body and my brain?

For the most part though, Dr. Marsh's questions confused me, and none of my answers seemed to fit perfectly. I second-guessed every word. Did I really choose to shop in smaller stores because I'm overwhelmed in large stores, or was it because smaller stores usually have cuter things? Did I really dislike being touched or was that only during anxiety attacks, when sensory input overwhelms me? *Which is it? How do I answer?* I could have spent an hour picking apart each question, looking at them from every angle, trying to find the truth amid the endless possibilities.

"Just give it your best guess," Dr. Marsh said, when I expressed my fears.

Later, she told me, "It's a very autistic thing to question the questions. Most neurotypical people don't sit around agonizing over whether they might be autistic." Meaning the agonizing itself was part of it.

At the end of our first session, I asked, "Do you need my parents to answer anything?"

During Delia's assessment, her mom had needed to complete a separate questionnaire to address what Delia was like as a child. It was the part of the assessment I dreaded the most. I still hadn't told anybody what I was doing, especially my parents, fully expecting another dismissal along the lines of "Yeah, but that's all normal. Everyone feels this way sometimes."

"You're welcome to get their help on the childhood section if you want," Dr. Marsh told me. "In order to qualify as autistic, symptoms need to have been present by the time you were three. But you don't need to involve your parents. I trust your memories and interpretations of them."

I stilled.

I trust your memories and interpretations of them.

For two years this phrase has repeated in my head. Every time I've questioned myself, I've rolled it around like a tumbled stone in my pocket. I recently called Dr. Marsh to ask her about this, still disbelieving that one's interpretation of themselves could be accurate. She was animated as she talked, clearly passionate about this question.

"The people I work with remember their own childhoods!" she said. "I give people the respect of believing them when they tell me what it was like. Plus, parents only see you from the outside; they don't know what's going on inside. If someone wants to give me input from a parent or sibling, I will certainly do that, but I don't require it. I don't say, 'I can't identify autism unless I talk to your mother.' I mean, I've assessed people in their sixties—their parents might not be living. And for some people, their parents are in denial." She paused, and I could feel her looking at me through the screen. "I want to level the playing field and get rid of as many barriers as possible."

At thirty-four years old, someone was at last telling me, *I believe you. I trust you. The way you see yourself matters.*

I stared at the Zoom window, but instead of my eyes wandering across the souvenirs on Dr. Marsh's desk, I glanced at the curled-up reflection of myself in the top right corner of the screen. Bags under my eyes, frizzy bun on top of my head, an unraveling knit blanket pulled up to my shoulders. I resisted the urge to look away.

THE FRIDAY OF OUR second interview, I was on the Oregon coast with some new friends. June and her buddy Sam were sharing a bunk bed and could be heard screaming throughout the house, arguing over who would get the top bunk. Andrea and I were attempting to work, while the dads had taken the day off and were planning to drag all three children to the beach. Even though the house we'd rented in Netarts Bay was chaos, and it definitely would have been better to take this appointment at home while June was at school so I wouldn't have to juggle work and vacation and screaming kids, there was no chance I was rescheduling, even by a week. Every day that passed without an answer was a day the word *autism* embedded itself more deeply in my soul. I'm not sure what I would have done had Dr. Marsh tried to pry it away.

"All right, I'm going downstairs for my appointment," I said to Elliot.

He squeezed my hand as I passed. "Good luck."

There wasn't anywhere comfortable and private for our second interview, so I propped myself in the queen bed, my back against the wall, trying to keep the wheeled mattress from rolling away. To my left, a sliding window overlooked the other condos surrounding the bay, and across the street, I could see a sliver of gray ocean, choppy in the wind. The muffled yell of a seagull filtered into the room.

I was less nervous this time, but my teeth chattered anyway as I clicked the Zoom link and waited for Dr. Marsh to arrive.

Once she logged on, we reviewed my next batch of survey responses and I fiddled with the string on my hoodie. I flared my nostrils, blinked my eyes hard, rolled my neck. The less I hid, the more I knew she could really see me.

At the end of our hour, surveys completed, all questions answered, I waited for whatever came next.

"Now that I have everything I need," she said, "I'll pull it into a report, which will have my findings and suggestions for accommodations, things like that."

"Great. Sounds good." I rolled my hoodie string into a tight spiral, then released it so it sprang away.

Was she going to say it? Was it implied? Would I have to wait until our final appointment when she walked me through the report? Would I have to wait another month? Was it inappropriate to ask her now whether I was or wasn't autistic?

While I debated whether to ask point-blank, she spoke again.

"Everything you've said to me lines up with a diagnosis. So yes, I believe you are autistic."

"Okay," I said, exhaling a gust of hot air I'd been holding for the past month. "Okay."

We said goodbye, and I closed the lid of my laptop and let it rest warm in my lap. I stared at the closet door, which was open a crack, and the lack of symmetry made the hairs on my arms stand up.

The house was quiet, so the kids must have left for the beach.

I texted Elliot. It's official. Autistic—I debated which emoji could possibly capture what I was feeling, but eventually I typed a final period and clicked Send.

I leaned my head against the wall and stared at the dusty ceiling.

Autistic.

The girls in fourth grade, cornering me in a closet for being too weird.

No, autistic.

Watching my best friends wrestle on the floor while I stood rooted behind the couch thinking, *What is wrong with you, what is wrong with you, what is wrong with you?*

Nothing. Autistic.

In college, quivering between days in bed, never brushing my teeth or hair or getting dressed for class, and copying Ami's every outfit and mannerism, hoping that if I looked normal on the outside, it would seep into my pores and change my genetic coding.

Autistic.

At work, trying to endure the office noise and chaos until I ran into the bathroom: lazy and worthless.

No, autistic.

I rubbed my face with my palms, trying to erase the decades of stories I'd been telling myself.

I rolled off the creaky bed, shut the closet door as I passed, and climbed the stairs. The rental was an upside-down condo with the living room and kitchen on top and a massive wall of windows that looked out over the bay. It was cold on the coast, and I could see our collective children on the beach, bracing against the wind. Andrea, my new and still-tender friend, was on the couch, editing wedding photos for a client.

She looked up when I entered.

"You autistic?" she asked.

One of my favorite things about Andrea, and the reason I've somehow managed to keep her for more than a year, is that she's clear in everything she says, and she seems to appreciate the nonsense that comes out of my mouth. Obviously, I was the same person I'd been that morning, but as I stood before her it occurred to me that this was a moment I could be with someone, not as their reflection or a performance of myself, but as Marian, autistic person. The mask I'd been wearing was starting to peel around the edges like old nail polish.

"Yup," I said, flopping on the couch across from her.

"You feel any different?"

I looked out the window at the out-of-place log cabin across the street, the strip of sand beyond and the angry waves beyond that. Elliot, Taylor, and the kids were walking back toward the condo.

"I don't know yet," I said, shaking my head. "I already knew. In my bones, ya know? I knew the moment I watched Delia's video, but it feels good to have a professional validate me instead of brushing me off."

Huh. How curious. The most revelatory moment came before I told anyone, before a doctor confirmed it, before I researched or read a word. The answer really had come from within.

The downstairs door opened, then slammed shut. What sounded like an army of raccoons tore inside, the house filled with footsteps and yelling. Two seconds later, June and Sam and Elliot and Taylor—baby Benny strapped to his chest—appeared upstairs, sandy and windswept. We wrangled our accumulated children, cleaned jellied hands, yelled "PLEASE SHARE" over our shoulders while navigating the stops and starts of conversation. I microwaved hot dogs while June and Sam argued over who would get to play on the iPad.

By early evening I was desperate for alone time, so I snuck outside to play with my new toy: an inflatable kayak I'd purchased off Craigslist and heaved out of a twentysomething's trunk in a Starbucks parking lot.

After fifteen minutes wrestling my inflated Goliath, I managed to fit all the pieces together and carry it over my shoulder to the beach, the wind pushing the front and tail ends, making me stumble through the sand.

The beach was empty this late in the day, and thank god, because it took seven tries to even get into the boat. The water was moving too fast, and the wind kept blowing the kayak from under me before I could hop in. On my first attempt, the kayak sailed past me and I fell straight into the water, soaking my leggings. I tried not to imagine the people in the beachfront houses looking out their windows and laughing.

I honestly couldn't tell you how I got in, but somehow the squeaky plastic supported my body, and with the shove of an oar, I pushed away from the shallow sand. The wind yanked me forward and I was flying.

The sun was low and glinting off the water. In the distance, I watched the silhouette of a woman standing on a paddleboard and a crab boat bobbing near a small island. What had been a colorless and blustery day turned pink and orange and red. The water shifted from gray to silver, like the underbelly of a fish. I paddled around to the far curve of the bay, where it opened to the ocean and the waves turned menacing.

I turned around to head home when two feet beyond my kayak, a whiskered brown face popped above the surface. A harbor seal! I *love* seals. They look like mermaid puppies. I've spent countless hours at the water's edge, scanning the surface for a glimpse of their round heads.

I stopped paddling and let the kayak drift so I could watch her, those big round eyes meeting mine. I looked back, steady. Clear pearls of water clung to her whiskers.

Two feet from her, another head appeared. Then another. And another.

Four seals seemingly appeared from nowhere and surrounded my boat, bobbing and unblinking. I gripped my plastic oar and swallowed. I imagined hundreds of seals below me, creatures I

couldn't see but who existed nonetheless, butting the hull from below, knocking me into the water and dragging me into the deep.

Yet I wasn't afraid.

I was no longer alone.

There were others like me here on earth, propelling themselves
through the world under a different type of steam. They were not
always visible to the naked eye, but it was comforting to know they
were there at all.

This whole time.

This whole time I thought I was broken. I'd wasted so much life
trying to pick up the shrapnel, slicing my fingers in the process, trying
to mosaic myself into the shape of a human, and now suddenly, with
a word, I was whole. Another creature entirely.

I stayed with the seals for as long as they would have me, until,
one by one, they disappeared under the water, and I paddled back
to shore.

—18—

A New Rule

"COME ON, PEANUT, *please* SIT DOWN."

Two weeks after my diagnosis, I stood on the curb next to June's preschool, facing the open door of our messy Prius, waiting for her to climb into her car seat. Behind us, a line of near-identical SUVs were in various stages of clown car. It was 5 p.m., but the temperature had just hit ninety and the sun beat on the pavement, not quite ready to relinquish its hold on the day. I leaned my forehead against the scalding doorframe.

"Mommy, can we listen to *Frozen II*?" June was no closer to sitting in her car seat, but she was standing *next* to it, draping the straps over her shoulders like panels on a clergy robe.

"Yes, fine. But sit down." Sweat beaded between my shoulder blades.

"Where does Elsa live?"

"In Arendelle, I think. Now *come on*."

June hopped into her seat, and I pounced in beside her to fasten the seventeen buckles that made up her Air Force jet harness. I tugged the tightening strap, panting.

"Mommy, are you angry?"

"No, baby, just hot. I get cranky when I'm hot."

"Is it my fault?"

My heart splintered. My biggest fear was that June would have to tiptoe around my moods, constantly trying to avoid triggering a meltdown, taking on the blame and responsibility when the problem was always me. It was too hot to dwell on my anxieties for long, though. So, so hot. The all-black car interior was suffocating, and the sensation of sweat snaking down my back took all the concentration I had away from being a pleasant parent. All I could think about was getting home.

"No, honey. It's not your fault. You are a perfect angel baby and I love you." I kissed her forehead and hightailed it to the front seat. I was lowering the temperature on the air-conditioning when she perked up from the back, her voice a gunshot.

"Mommy, *Frozen*!"

"Yes, honey, *I know*. Give me two seconds, I literally just turned on the car." The tone that came out of me was not the tone I'd intended. I'd planned to be all tranquil patience, like a mom from school whom I watched exit the main doors, hand in hand with her chattering, skipping daughter, nodding with a serenity I only ever experienced when I was alone.

I scrambled to connect my phone to Bluetooth and start the *Frozen II* soundtrack before June could nag again. I dreaded the unpredictability of her requests. I knew they were coming, but I never knew when, so my shoulders slid toward my neck and my whole body tensed. The anticipation was worse than the sound itself.

Idina Menzel's voice filled the car. June was mostly quiet when music played, and I can't lie, the *Frozen II* soundtrack is fire.

"Mommy, your favorite song!"

"I know. I *love* this song."

We pulled away from the school and onto Thirty-Third Avenue. Traffic wasn't too bad, but there was construction on the corner, and making a left around the cones always made me jittery. I turned down the music so I could see better.

"Mommy, I can't heeear!" June whined.

My tires squealed as I made the turn, right as the light flicked to red, just as the blue car opposite us blasted through the final second of his yellow and then, almost gently, like two spinning ballerinas, we careened around each other in a perfect, death-defying arc. Neither of us honked, but I could feel the near miss in my teeth.

"Mommy, louder!"

I turned the music back up without thinking, so used to doing whatever is asked of me, even from a four-year-old, even as my vision tunneled and my pulse traveled to the base of my throat.

I have always been a fortress
Cold secrets deep inside

"Where is Elsa's mommy?" June asked from the back seat.

I could barely make out her question over the music. My mind started to spin with an answer a child could understand. *Her mom is dead, but why is she singing in this song? Is she a ghost? If she's a ghost, why can't Elsa talk to her? Was the voice Elsa's mom or the fifth spirit, and if Elsa is the fifth spirit, was she calling to herself this whole time?*

I'm sure this took only a split second, but I was waiting for another question, another interruption, so I reached for a fast answer that wouldn't lead to ten thousand more questions and my heart was still racing from the near-accident and the music was burrowing in my ear like an angry groundhog and—

The words *SHUT UP SHUT UP SHUT UP* appeared at the pit of my stomach, a bull stomping his feet and ready for the gate to spring open so he could race out of there, dust flying behind him.

Wait, whispered a voice.

The world slowed and a new wire connected in my brain, the prongs of an abandoned extension cord fitting into an outlet labeled AUTISM.

This is the start of a meltdown.

I didn't open the gate.

Instead, I reached over six inches and paused the music. The car filled with silence and relief.

"I need a second, June."

I took a right onto the next street, pulled over, and put the car in park.

"Are we taking a different way?" June asked.

"Please give me a second."

I closed my eyes. *You are not broken*, I told myself. *You're autistic. There's a lot of stimulation happening right now; it makes total sense that you'd snap. You're okay. June can wait for you to regulate.*

When I finally did, I unbuckled my seat belt and turned around to look at my beautiful, patient daughter.

"No, honey, we're not taking a different way. I need to talk to you."

"Okay."

"We need a new rule." I paused. Ten thousand thoughts raced through my head, and I searched for the right thread to pull, fully formed, without a hundred other tangents getting tangled up with it.

"You know how sometimes Mommy yells at you?"

"Yes. You need to use your words."

"Exactly. Which is what I'm doing right now. Back at school, I said the heat was making me a little cranky. Then I was driving, and the driving was making me a little cranky. Then the music was too loud, and I really really wanted to yell. It's not your fault. It's not your fault *at all*. I have something called autism."

"What's autism?"

"Autism is just a different way my brain works. You know how at school you're learning about all the different skin colors people have?"

"Yes. We have peachy skin."

"That's right. And sometimes you and I talk about how people come in different sizes. Like how Daddy has a flat tummy, but Mommy has a round tummy."

"I have a little tummy!"

"You do! Well, autism is kind of like that, except it's inside people's brains, so you can't always see it from the outside. But it means that some things, especially noises, can make my brain confused. And if there are too many noises, or too many things that want my attention, I yell."

"Do I have autism?"

"I don't know, sweetheart."

"Mommy?"

"Yeah, baby?"

"Can you turn the music back on?"

I laughed. "In a minute. Here's the new rule. If you want to talk while I'm driving, we need to pause the music first. I can't answer any questions while music is playing."

"Okay!"

"And," I continued, "sometimes I *can't* talk when I'm driving, especially to answer complicated questions. I need to be extra careful and pay attention. It's dangerous to focus on you while also trying to get us home safely, so I might say, 'Hold on,' and you'll need to wait until I'm ready. Can you do that?"

"Yes."

I don't know how much she really heard me, but the air shifted in that moment. I could rebuild the world—for myself.

"All right, let's try this!" I clicked my seat belt back into place. "Thanks for listening, kiddo." As I pulled into the road again, Idina Menzel came back on and I swear to god if that line *You are the one you've been waiting for all of your life* didn't blast through the speakers at that exact second.

While the song played, we headed back for home, my heart no longer pounding under my skin, crawling up my belly and into my chest, threatening to burst all over the people I loved. I drove through the leafy Portland streets, past the mansions of Laurelhurst and the half-built condos on Burnside, as June's high little-girl voice sang along in the back seat.

UNTIL THAT REVELATION IN the car with June, I'd never truly given myself permission to ask for what I needed. I lived by an arduous, ever-growing list of rules based on what I thought "normal people" did. If I ever fell short, I bullied myself into normalcy: *Why can't you just _____ ?*

When I inevitably melted down or retreated into myself, I assumed I wasn't trying hard enough. It's not that I *couldn't* listen to music while talking to my kid and driving, it's that I *didn't want it bad enough*.

Turns out, I could change the rules.

It took practice, of course. June would start talking, and I'd say, "Hang on, let me turn off the music." Then I'd ask, "Okay, what did you want to say?" And she'd ask questions about why birds fly or how old I'll be when she's nineteen or whether Elsa's castle is at Disneyland, and I answered them without noise competing for my mental attention.

And I just . . . stopped yelling.

Over the following weeks and months, this new way of being flowed into every area of my life. I discovered my triggers, then slowly and methodically removed them.

"June, we can talk or watch the movie, I can't do both."

"Honey, I'm trying to focus on writing this text right now, and I can't concentrate while you're talking to me. Give me two minutes to finish and then I can answer your question."

And it wasn't only June, it was everyone. How had I never noticed how much people multitask? They talk while writing text messages, work while listening to a podcast, and have long and lingering conversations in coffee shops while pop music screeches through the wall speakers. How had I never noticed how much the sensory experience of the world was splitting me apart?

I can't I can't I can't.

There was so much freedom in *can't*.

The autism community is split on this. Some autistic people believe phrases like "She just can't help it" are infantilizing, while others have found space and compassion in understanding the borders of their tolerance. Knowing my brain is physically wired in this particular way has allowed me to stop fiddling with the cables and just let them be.

I've interviewed and read accounts from hundreds of late-diagnosed autistic people, and each one articulated the same idea: once they learned the name for how they show up in the world, there was space to think, change their environment, and forgive themselves for all the ways they had thought they were broken.

Artist and musician Morgan Harper Nichols learned she was autistic in her thirties. She wrote a blog post expressing gratitude for language that explains her way of moving through the world: "I can honestly say this experience of getting diagnosed has ultimately left me feeling supported and like I have permission to breathe just a little bit more, knowing that there are explanations for my experiences and the struggles I face."

Once we can breathe, there's space leftover to figure out what we need. We might never change, but our environment can. Hannah Gadsby articulated this perfectly in their memoir, *Ten Steps to Nanette*. "Once I understood that I was always going to have difficulty with self-regulation, I stopped worrying about it. Once I am distressed, my moods are not mine to control, but my environment is . . . I have learned how to advocate for my own experiences instead of being ashamed of my pain and confusion."

Which brings me to Step Three on the Path to Autistic Self-Actualization: once we're breathing and adapting our environment to suit our needs, we can forgive. When Dr. Marsh told me about the patients she's assessed over the years, she said, "You know that quote by Maya Angelou? 'Do the best you can until you know better. Then when you know better, do better'? I think that quote says it for a lot of people. They say to me, 'Now I can forgive my teachers and my parents and myself. We did not know better then, but now we do.'"

Maia Szalavitz wrote about autism and forgiveness in an essay for *Matter*. "I thought I was incapable of relationships and irreparably damaged. If I had received the diagnosis, I might have at least understood that there were other people like me, that it wasn't my fault."

Not my fault.

I couldn't try my way out of this. I couldn't meditate or gratitude journal or breathe my way into being a real person. I already was a real person, and learning that fact felt like crawling into a crisp hotel bed after a lifetime of sleeping upright in a barn. I could forgive myself for leaving early, ending friendships, speaking bluntly, asking for clarification, covering my ears, forgoing a bra, locking my knees, retreating to dark spaces, watching too much TV, reading the diary, running from the cockroach, yelling at my daughter—and eventually, I would never blame myself at all.

Diagnosis code F84.0 changed my parenting, my relationships, and my career, in so many ways that snowballed into a life I no longer recognized. A month or so after my *Frozen*-inspired car epiphany, I had a meeting with a few of my coworkers. We had these a couple of times per week, a group of us writing together in one big Google Doc. When the time came to log on to Zoom, I sat at my desk to ensure the best view of my office. I noticed my bun was falling over to the side, so I quickly retied it before clicking Join. Tanya and Liz and Alice and Kat and Steffi were already settled, their little boxes revealing entire worlds I needed to decipher.

Is Liz in a bad mood? Why is Alice looking away from her computer?

Kat always looks so put together: Doesn't she have like five kids? Steffi's the only one smiling: Do I need to smile back? Will I look grumpy if I don't? I checked my face in the self view. *Uh-oh, Tanya is asking me something, and shit, I forgot what this meeting was about . . .*

"Sorry, what?" I asked. I grabbed a nail polish bottle from my desk and started rolling it in my palms.

"Can you loop us in on how the program scripts are going for Module 1?" she said.

"Ah, right." I put down the bottle and opened Google Drive, trying to find my folder with the scripts. *Why do I never prepare for meetings?* I stalled for time. "Yeah, they're, um, going . . ."

For a long, painful minute I stuttered through my update while also trying to read everyone's facial expressions while also worrying about my own while also getting philosophical about eye contact. *Why does digital eye contact feel exactly the same as real eye contact? I'm not looking at their actual eyes.* Which is when the voice in my head spoke up for the hundredth time that fall (she was getting louder now): *Hello! Marian! You are autistic. There is too much stimulation right now. There is literally nothing you can do to behave the way they do. Change your environment.*

"Hang on," I interrupted myself. "I'm going to turn off my video if you don't mind. I'm finding it distracting."

Oh no no no, take it back, what have you done?

"Dude, do what you gotta do," said Tanya.

I turned off my video and minimized Zoom and in an instant, like a literal light switch, I could think again. I gave a seamless, articulate update. I listened thoughtfully, then asked smart questions. I was more fully myself when I wasn't trying to read the room and talk at the same time. And the best part is . . . no one cared. Not a single one! In fact, Alice turned off her camera a few minutes after I did and messaged me later to say, "Thanks! I hate video calls too." I felt like a pioneer. Is this what it's like to be a man?

At work, I became the Person Who Doesn't Go on Camera.

Sometimes I turned it on for a second to say hi and prove that I wasn't half listening on a beach in Bali, but I'd always say, "Okay, I'm going to turn this off again." Sometimes it sparked a conversation about how video calls are distracting, but most of the time, no one commented.

On another night, my new friend Harper invited me to a book reading. When I arrived at Powell's, it was standing room only. For about thirty seconds I stood in the back, which was getting hotter and stuffier by the second. Old Marian would have stayed for the whole event because she thought she had to, because this is what people in their thirties do, and she would have grown more and more resentful as the minutes ticked down. By the time it was over, she would have been unrecognizable—a curt, rude mess—to this perky blonde she had met at knit night and probably ended the friendship before it had a chance to start.

Instead, an understanding hit me, with all the force of a speeding train: *I don't need to suffer through this anymore.*

I texted Harper, who I'd told about my diagnosis soon after we met. I'm gonna go! Too much sensory stuff, sorry. Had no idea this would be so popular. Have fun!

I drove home, got into bed, and ate sour candy while watching *SNL* clips on YouTube.

An entirely new world opened up to me, one with boundaries and self-compassion and honest relationships. My diagnosis gave me permission to honor what my brain needed. A lifetime of "pushing through" and negative self-talk and guilt and shame was just . . . over.

—19—

Impostor

"I HOPE YOU SPEND AS MUCH TIME ADVOCATING FOR REAL DISABILITY rights as you do broadcasting your diagnosis."

"The spectrum should remain subject to strict guidelines. Doing otherwise takes away from the severity of the symptoms and treatments needed for real autistic people."

"So you get to be cute and married, well-traveled, brilliant, an accomplished and published writer for prestigious publications . . . a MOTHER (which is what my daughter and her autistic female friends dream of but will likely never be) . . . AND a part of the autism club? Why do you get to be at the top of the functioning autism spectrum? Where does that leave other people with autism? Where does that leave my daughter?"

Well, shit.

Two weeks earlier, I'd been reading my favorite blog, *Cup of Jo*, when I saw that the editor had linked to an essay by Hannah Gadsby about their autism diagnosis. I beamed at the sight of my worlds colliding: the woman I always wanted to be dissolving to make way for the woman I'd always been—a piece of me reflected in this aspirational muted-pink lifestyle website. I scrolled down to the comments and wrote a quick, delighted note about my own

diagnosis and how thrilled I was to see myself represented somewhere so mainstream.

A few days later, a woman named Iris also left a glowing comment about the Hannah Gadsby inclusion, along with a request to
the editor, "Sometime this month, please consider sharing more stories from #actuallyautistic people. We need to counter the messages
of stigma and shame, and work to create a culture that celebrates,
accepts, and embraces Autistic folks so this generation of kids can
grow up with the understanding and support they need!"

I hadn't written a personal essay in years, but as I read Iris's comment, an idea began to take shape, a fizzing sensation along my skin.
What if I shared my *story?* Writing had always been my preferred way
to connect, so why not now? Why not about this?

Without thinking too long or hard about it, I emailed the editor,
Joanna: Did she want me to write about my experience of living undiagnosed for thirty-four years, and about how drastically my life had
changed in the six months since I'd learned I'd been autistic all along?

Two hours later, my inbox displayed a new message. "Oh my
gosh, yes!" she'd written back. "We would absolutely love a piece on
this topic, which is near and dear to my heart."

That week, in the quiet dark of the mornings before work, I wrote
about the closet in fourth grade, about Lewis and his friends in that
London bar, and about the sensory overload of parenting. As I wrote,
I ached to hold the nine- and twenty-two- and thirty-one-year-old
versions of me who ran sobbing out of bars and flung her possessions
into walls, feeling like the loneliest, angriest person in the world. I
had let very few people see these parts of myself, and it felt like shed-
ding layers of my mask onto the page.

Yet, on the day of publication, my stomach roiled with dread.

What did I *really* know about autism? I'd understood this side
of myself for only six months. I wasn't a researcher or a doctor or a
scientist. What if I said something wrong? What if no one believed
me? My self-compassion was still tenuous, so I vowed not to read

the comments in case the internet decided to do what the internet does best.

I tried—I really did try—to accept that sharing my story was enough. Why hunt for reasons to doubt myself?

For weeks after my essay's publication, I stayed strong, but I felt like a sixth grader in the cafeteria, hearing the popular girls whisper while giving me the side-eye, knowing they were gossiping about me but unable to make out their words.

A month or so later, I gave into the itch to eavesdrop. I scrolled below my bio to "201 comments," squared my shoulders, and started to read.

My instincts had been right. The top comment was from "Margie," who'd clearly had enough of whatever bloody massacre had happened below.

> *There are many things I would like to say to the surprisingly large amount of people on here saying that, essentially, because my son is verbal, he isn't disabled enough to be autistic, or need services, or deserve the same advocacy as a more deserving (wtaf) autistic person, but I am so upset I can't really form thoughts. . . .*

Oh boy oh boy oh boy. I swallowed the sour burn that had traveled up my throat, then scrolled farther.

The next few comments were lovely—dozens of autistic women who weren't diagnosed until their thirties, forties, and even fifties. For decades they'd been told, "You're just anxious" and "Try harder. Make more friends. Put yourself out there." And when the women who knew that autism can look different from the stereotypes were brave enough to ask, their doctors had said, "You can't be autistic; it's a boys' disorder."

Dozens more women shared that they'd been diagnosed with ADHD, OCD, sensory processing disorders, even endometriosis after years of searching for an answer. They'd always been over-whelmed and alienated, "a little off." Getting a diagnosis was a light in the darkness.

With each positive comment, I paused to fill my tank for what I knew was coming. *Thank you*, I replied to each of them. *Thank you for seeing me.*

Then I got to the girls in the cafeteria.

If someone has autism, they actually wouldn't be able to speak for themselves, or live any sort of typical life. There needs to be a different name for people who have "asperger-type" character-istics. It is very, very difficult to see someone who has a mostly normal life be put in the same category as my son, who has needed constant attention and supervision and special care since he was a baby, and requires every single thing in our daily lives to take him into consideration.

I take issue with the use of the term autism. Why isn't calling it neurodiverse enough for someone high functioning? To use the term autism for what the author describes just really feels like coopting a vulnerable category. If everything means anything, nothing means anything.

I would argue that we need to do away with the idea that any-one is "neurotypical." We all struggle with different aspects of functionality in society. Finding a diagnosis may bring some peace, but I don't think anyone feels particularly "normal." Furthermore, please give some consideration to taking on the label of disability when one is able to move without restriction through an ableist society.

Each dismissal flung me off some high cliff, my stomach plum-meting to my toes before lurching back up again. I struggled to control my breathing, but it came out fast and shallow. My jaw locked and my bones shook.

How could I possibly have thought this was a good idea? I *knew* I'd been trying to claim an identity that wasn't mine.

Hundreds of positive comments couldn't insulate me from the dozen or so eviscerating ones that spoke to every fear and doubt I'd ever had. It didn't matter that not a single critical comment came from someone who was *actually autistic*—a phrase I later learned is used to counter assumptions that primarily come from caregivers and not autistic people themselves—all I heard was the mob of outraged parents who had "worse" autistic kids, yelling outside my door.

I closed my computer, then my eyes. I placed a hand on my heart and felt its steady beat. I was still alive, somehow, but I had traveled back in time to Mr. Bacon's fourth-grade closet and was cowering behind a ski jacket while the girls on the other side told me to shut up, stop talking, stop taking up space.

What was I thinking?

Does having this diagnosis mean I'm taking resources from someone else?

Does sharing my story make more "severe" autism less meaningful?

What if Dr. Marsh got it wrong?

A MONTH AFTER MY diagnosis, I'd joined an online group with over ten thousand autistic women. After reading the comments on my essay, it was the only place I could think to turn for clarity. Still in bed, I sighed and cracked open my computer again.

On the group's discussion board, I typed, "For those of you who've been officially diagnosed with ASD—specifically later in life—do you ever feel like, 'My doctor must be wrong?' Have you ever questioned your diagnosis? The autistic label has been so helpful for me this year, and at the same time I can't help feeling like an impostor."

Within minutes I had to mute my computer because of the *bing! bing! bing!* of notifications.

"I can identify with this," wrote a woman named Lucinda. "I have wondered if my answers have been swayed by wanting to finally feel like I fit in somewhere, and that perhaps I'm just an impostor and don't belong at all."

Another woman named Meike wrote, "Keep in mind that representation, especially when it comes to autism, is almost always reinforcing stereotypes because a) it sells well and b) people can relate to this version of autism because it's all they're being told. The majority of autistic people are people you wouldn't recognize as autistic if you met them on the street."

And when I parroted back an angry mom (and Dr. Anderson) who claimed that because I was married and well-traveled and a writer and mother, I couldn't possibly be autistic, Miranda reminded me, "What you have in life doesn't really have anything to do with whether or not you have ASD. I have a successful career and my own home and family too, but I'm definitely on the spectrum."

A commenter named Heather chimed in, "I don't see anyone saying the same thing to Elon Musk."

Over and over these women repeated, "We all went through this impostor phase. It's okay, you're still one of us." My shoulders softened.

And yet, one pesky comment stayed lodged in my mind. I kept returning to the blog to read it again and again, trying to wrap my head around her words. The anonymous commenter (I know, I know) claimed to be a psychologist who specializes in fixing incorrect diagnoses. She said, sympathetically, that just because someone meets criteria on a checklist, it doesn't mean they match with the underlying "gestalt" of a complete diagnosis. "The level of social insight you present with sounds a bit in contradiction to the inherent

diagnostic gestalt of Autism," she wrote. "You may have sensory processing difficulties, social-communication disorder, ADHD, anxiety,
or a combo issue of the above. I would love for you to get a second
opinion just to be sure."

Looking back, I have no idea why this comment burrowed in
my psyche like a splinter, but I couldn't stop picking at it. She wasn't
angry or devastated by a child's struggle; she was coherent and kind.
In fact, her comment made a lot of sense. I might not be *great*
with people, but I'm emotive and empathetic and well-spoken. I'm
not completely clueless about human beings and their experiences.
Didn't that go against everything that made autism *autism*? The
deep, terrifying truth inside me was that, even after six months of
life-changing shifts in my mental health, and even with the support
and camaraderie of other autistic women, I did wonder whether I
was *really* autistic. Could I have wanted an answer from Dr. Marsh
so urgently that I somehow led the witness? Plus, if a handful of
internet comments could bring it all crashing down, how real could
my diagnosis be?

THE ONLY WAY TO silence the doubt was a second opinion.

Back when I'd done my first round of frantic internet research,
one name popped up in all the blogs and videos: a British author
named Sarah Hendrickx. Sarah is a world-renowned expert who's
worked with autistic people for decades and wrote the classic book
Women and Girls on the Autism Spectrum. She's English, which is why
I hadn't considered working with her for my first assessment, but
this time the thought was comforting. I'd had an easier time living
outside America—of course my second opinion should come from
England.

I messaged Sarah's team and woke up the next day to an email
from her husband, Keith. "Prior to booking," he wrote, "we suggest
taking the following tests to be sure that an Autism assessment is

right for you in order to save your time and money. You are welcome to share your scores and we can give our opinion." He linked me to two tests: the Autism Spectrum Quotient (AQ) and the Camouflaging Autistic Traits Questionnaire (CAT-Q).

Since you can't verify autism with a blood test or a brain scan, the diagnostic processes can be as varied as their providers. Delia's diagnosis involved a series of in-person psychiatrist appointments and a survey completed by her parents. Dr. Marsh relies on a combination of standard tests and questionnaires of her own creation. Sarah Hendrickx uses two online screening tests followed by a long-form written questionnaire and an interview.

I'd taken the AQ the previous year, but I'd never heard of the CAT-Q, a questionnaire developed in 2018 by Dr. Laura Hull, currently at the University of Bristol, to measure social camouflaging behaviors in adults. These behaviors can be used to identify autistic people who don't meet diagnostic criteria because they've spent so long trying to *hide* their autistic traits.

The AQ and the CAT-Q are by no means the only psychometric tests available. There's the Aspie Quiz, which indicates whether someone is neurodivergent, neurotypical, or mixed; the Empathy Quotient, which tests the ability to tune in to how someone else is feeling; and the RBQ-2A, which measures restricted and repetitive behaviors. Turns out, there's more than one way to skin a cockroach.

I found the CAT-Q on the website Embrace Autism, run by Natalie Engelbrecht, a naturopathic doctor, psychotherapist, and researcher in Canada. Natalie spent years collecting all the major diagnostic questionnaires, then turned them into easy-to-take online tests that will automatically calculate your scores. She gave each questionnaire a rating based on testing accuracy, respectful language, and clarity, and she even includes discussion notes where she and her team share their own results, making you feel like you're learning about yourself in community with other autistics.

On the CAT-Q, Natalie wrote, "I like that the CAT-Q addresses some of the problems with the outdated definitions of autism in the research literature. It can also identify a person with autism who might score below the threshold of other autism tests due to Masking. I scored 143, which is significantly higher than most autistic females (124), and autistics in general. That is not a surprise as I have always camouflaged so much that therapists never diagnosed me with autism until age 47."

I sent my results back to Keith (I scored a whopping 146 on the CAT-Q), and he responded that both my AQ and CAT-Q were within the range expected for an autistic person, and an assessment with Sarah would likely be informative. I didn't tell Keith or Sarah about my previous diagnosis, hoping to get a fully unbiased second opinion.

By the time Sarah and I met on Zoom, it was late August, exactly a year after Dr. Marsh had diagnosed me.

For two and a half hours, Sarah and I laughed like old friends. It was different going through the assessment with an autistic person— more vulnerable and straightforward, less pressurized. At the two-hour mark Sarah and I were talking about friendships, and whether I *wanted* friends or felt their absence because I'm "supposed" to want them, when she abruptly switched gears.

"So what you do think?" she asked. "Do you think you're autistic?"

Caught off guard, I laughed. "Do *I* think I'm autistic?"

"Yeah." She was laughing too, as if it were obvious. It was obvious to me too, commenters be damned.

"I mean, yeah. I do." My voice was a shrug.

"Me too." She sighed and shook her head. "No doubt whatsoever. Not in the slightest."

"What makes you say that?" I asked.

"All of it," she said. "There is no one moment or response that leads to the autistic conclusion—it is the culmination of responses to all the questions. An autism diagnosis is a package of cognition, behaviors, and perceptions covering all aspects of the diagnostic criteria, so it can never be just one thing."

"You know, I wasn't going to tell you this, but I was diagnosed last year," I admitted.

She startled. "With autism?"

"Yeah."

I explained the story of my diagnosis, the essay, the comments. I talked and talked, spilling my impostor syndrome at Sarah's feet.

"Where was this essay published?" she interrupted. "In the US?"

"Yeah, on an American site."

"That would be the first thing that comes to mind. The US is quite a long way behind in terms of adults and in terms of women. I came to the States maybe four or five years ago to speak at a big autism conference. Temple Grandin was headlining, thousands of people in attendance. And look, I'm quite well-known, I've written a lot of books, but only fourteen people showed up to my session. Out of three *thousand* delegates. No one cared to talk about women at all. Whereas over here, in the UK, you can fill an entire conference just talking about autistic women."

"Wow. I had no idea."

"It's also my understanding that the parent brigade is much more militant in the US. There's a real battle between autistic adults and people with autistic children."

I was nodding like a bobblehead. Even that made sense. American disability services are a joke, so caregivers have to be militant if they want to make their children's lives easier.

"You also have to remember that a lot of these parents are autistic themselves," Sarah continued. "It's highly genetic. These are autistic people with autistic children. That's the great irony! They're rigid! They think they're right!"

"Oh my god!" I shouted, thinking of my own father, who I had started suspecting was autistic nearly ten years prior. "Why did that never occur to me?"

Over the following months, I devoured everything I could about the parent brigade's main arguments, which boiled down to one simple objection: *Your autism doesn't look like the autism I know.*

The more I read, the more I realized our differences centered on a single misused word. As it turns out, we've been using *spectrum* all wrong.

AS A WRITER, I'M embarrassed I didn't realize this myself. I thought *spectrum* meant *range*. *I'm on the spectrum* meant yes, I have a developmental disorder, but it's not immediately obvious to people on the street, so that means I'm on the mild end of the spectrum, while other people can and do have it more severely.

Turns out, that's a *gradient*. A spectrum is something else entirely.

The best piece of writing on this topic is C. L. Lynch's 2019 essay at NeuroClastic, "'Autism Is a Spectrum' Doesn't Mean What You Think." Lynch explains that referring to people as being "more" or "less" autistic is like comparing red to green, or apples to oranges. "Red isn't 'more spectrum' than green," she writes. "Apples aren't 'more fruit' than oranges." People can't be a little autistic or extremely autistic. There's no such thing as an autism ladder with me standing at the bottom and Dustin Hoffman counting toothpicks at the top. A spectrum is not a ranking of severity.

The autism spectrum is what the *DSM-5* calls an "uneven profile of abilities," a collection of related neurological conditions, *each one* presenting differently depending on the person.

"If you only check one or two boxes, then they don't call it autism—they call it something else," Lynch writes. "For example, if you ONLY struggle with communication, then they call that social communication disorder. If you ONLY have problems with body movement/control then that is called dyspraxia or developmental coordination disorder. If you ONLY have sensory processing issues then that is sensory processing disorder. But if you have all of the above and more, they call it autism."

Within each of those boxes, *then* there is a sort of gradient. One autistic person, Bob, may have large, noticeable repetitive behaviors that may seem distracting in a classroom setting, but he can go to a loud, bright bar with no problems. Another autistic person, Sarah, could be so sensitive to sound and light and touch that she walks around in public with headphones, sunglasses, and a fidget spinner, but she speaks verbally with easy eye contact. Who is more "severe"? Who is less "functional"?

It's also worth pointing out—*again*—that the definition of autism doesn't include intellectual disability or language impairment. The stereotype of someone with "severe autism" often includes one or more other conditions that can *co-occur* with autism, like epilepsy, intellectual disabilities, apraxia, or Ehlers-Danlos syndrome, but aren't technically part of autism itself.

In previous editions, the *DSM* split autism into three different diagnoses: autism, pervasive developmental disorder (PDD), and Asperger's syndrome. The latter was seen as the more "high-functioning," "intelligent" version of autism, and you may have heard it used to describe folks like Elon Musk or Greta Thunberg. But in 2013, with the publication of the *DSM-5*, Asperger's and PDD were both removed and effectively merged into a more holistic, encompassing diagnosis: autism spectrum disorder.

The differences between Asperger's and autism had always been murky, without much evidence to support a distinction between the two. Since autism was widely accepted as varied anyway, it didn't make a ton of sense to separate it into three categories. Of course, people were furious, terrified that the change in diagnosis might limit services for their children or change their own identity, since many people connected strongly with the term *aspie*. Francesca Happé, professor of cognitive neuroscience at King's College London and a member of the work group for the *DSM-5* rewrite, laid out her thinking in an article about their decision: "Should Asperger syndrome be re-defined as 'autism without accompanying intellectual or language deficits'? This is fine descriptively but makes no sense in terms of diagnosis; neither intellectual disability nor language impairment are part of the definition of autism."

Asperger's was named after Hans Asperger, the Austrian physician who's often credited with discovering the condition. For decades, he was considered a hero, claiming to have resisted the Nazis by saving disabled children during World War II. After his death, he was partially responsible for increasing awareness that autistic people can be intelligent and speak well. But in 2018, five years after the *DSM* change, historians Edith Sheffer and Herwig Czech separately published information linking Asperger to the Third Reich. He had sent dozens of children—what he called the most "difficult cases"—to Am Spiegelgrund, Vienna's "children's clinic" and killing center. His reputation never recovered.

Edith Sheffer has an autistic son, who'd been diagnosed with Asperger's before the *DSM* change, but Sheffer was supportive of the merger, despite its imperfections. "Hopefully, as research progresses, we will develop a more appropriate vocabulary," she wrote in *Scientific American*. "In the meantime, we can effect a positive change by no longer invoking Asperger's name."

Despite Asperger's falling out of fashion, you'll still hear autistic people described as "high functioning" or "low functioning," phrases referring to traits that hold societal value, like communicating verbally, socializing in person, and making contributions to a capitalist economy—traits that have nothing to do with someone's well-being or happiness. When we categorize people by their monetary value to society, we imply that "low-functioning" people are not worthy members of it.

This all assumes that functionality is even measurable. I may be employed, but I spent my first decade in corporate America sobbing in office bathrooms in order to stay that way. A nonspeaking autistic person may struggle during a job interview but crave highly complex, social work. Hari Srinivasan, a minimally speaking autistic, is a student earning his PhD in neuroscience at Vanderbilt, an alum of UC Berkeley, and has held fellowships at Paul and Daisy Soros Fellowships for New Americans, the OpEd Project, and the Frist Center for Autism and Innovation. He's also on six separate boards, including the Autistic Self Advocacy Network (ASAN) and the BRAIN Foundation. Hari perfectly summed up the problem with categorizing people by functionality in an email he sent me: "It's not a comparison. Disability looks different for each person, depending on intersectionality and other issues they are dealing with, and the environment they are in at that moment."

Many caregivers want to separate high-functioning and low-functioning autism for reasons that feel altruistic: What's more noble than fighting for your children? But by insisting on black-and-white distinctions, the caregivers may undermine the efforts they claim to champion. Why presume incompetence for "low-functioning" people if the goal is better accommodations and more dignity?

Which is why the second objection I heard was equally maddening: *No one is really normal! We all struggle. Stop labeling everything! Let's accept everyone for who they are.*

I mean, sure.

In a perfect world we'd all be free to be you and me. In a perfect world I could have asked for and received accommodations years ago without being called names. In a perfect world all disabled people would have equal opportunities and access to whatever supports enable us to participate in all areas of society. But we don't live in a perfect world, and it's cruel to decide that someone who's struggling should continue to struggle because a label makes you uncomfortable. For a student to receive services, they need a diagnosis. For a person to get benefits, they need a diagnosis. For an employee to qualify for office accommodations, they need—wait for it—a diagnosis.

Autistic people die significantly younger than neurotypicals, with one study showing an average life expectancy of thirty-nine years. One common reason for this high mortality is suicide, with rates *nine times* higher than neurotypicals. Nine. Times. Most autistic people who die by suicide are what people would call "high functioning," in that they were previously diagnosed with Asperger's or don't have co-occurring intellectual disabilities. So we should be fine, right? We're smart and functional and therefore can't possibly be disabled? The truth is, autistic children are almost six times more likely to consider suicide if they have an IQ of 120 or higher.

So functional. So much less severe.

Until that perfect world magically exists, what are we supposed to do? Spend our lives watching the rest of the world laugh in bars with their heads thrown back and get baby showers organized on their behalf and make it through a single day at work without a shrieking meltdown?

For better or worse, labels help us make sense of ourselves, help us understand our needs and our place in the world. Labels dull the ache of dismissal. Labels help us find community when we've spent most of our lives alone. Labels allow the people who love and care for us to do so more effectively.

Joanna Goddard, the editor of *Cup of Jo*, has a neurodivergent son. In response to one of these "free to be you and me" comments on my essay, she wrote,

> When I hear, "Oh, everyone would need help with that!" or, "All kids would benefit from services like that!" or, "But he seems so normal!" I feel completely misunderstood. We work so hard to get the right services and school programs and private schooling and neuropsychological evaluations and therapists and supports and medications and camps and even lawyers, since our neurodiverse kids truly cannot thrive in neurotypical school systems and settings (even when the schools are excellent) or make lasting friendships with neurotypical kids, and we have had

parenting challenges that are different from neurotypical parents
from the time our babies were just a few months old. We read a
gazillion books and talk to a gazillion experts and other parents
and get tough school feedback and try to figure out the systems
and paths forward, and clutch our hearts at night with love and
worry. So it feels dismissive of all that challenge and effort and
work and love when someone says, "Oh we're all in the same
boat."

Sometimes what people most need in these moments is to know that things *aren't* normal. If I had a word cloud for all my conversations with autistic women over the past two years, the biggest word would be *validated*. So no, we can't just embrace that we're all a little bit weird. Because if you're not autistic, you and I are not the same, and I'd rather have you acknowledge that difference than keep gaslighting me until I die. I am more similar to someone you think is "severely autistic" than I am to someone who is neurotypical. This analogy from autistic activist John Marble explains it best: "There's millions of different ways to be French, and a gay fashion designer in Paris and a Catholic nun in Bordeaux are going to be radically different. But they still understand each other as French."

And that includes autistic people who self-diagnose, not only people with a doctor's note. Because as much as I can harp on about the benefits of an official diagnosis, the reality is that getting one is extremely difficult. It's expensive as hell; very few psychiatrists and doctors specialize in masked presentation; and in our deeply ableist society, a diagnosis on paper may do more harm than good. For example, many countries won't allow an autistic person to immigrate, including my old home of New Zealand. In the United States, over half the states have policies that suggest people with cognitive disabilities would be deprioritized for ventilators in the event of a shortage. Disabled parents face frequent discrimination during divorce proceedings. My diagnosis could, theoretically, prevent me from getting custody of June in the event that Elliot turns into an asshole. Many late-identified autistic adults have decided to save the money and avoid a paper trail by self-diagnosing.

In *Unmasking Autism*, Devon Price writes that hearing from other autistic people was his true moment of power and self-acceptance, *not* the piece of paper that ultimately confirmed his suspicions.

> *These connections to the Autism self-advocacy world would end up doing far more for me than the psychological establishment did. Establishing official recognition of my disability was challenging, bureaucratic, and ultimately felt very hollow and meaningless—much like getting legal recognition of my gender. I was Autistic long before any professional recognized it, just as I was trans long before the state acknowledged it . . . Diagnosis is a gatekeeping process, and it slams its heavy bars in the face of anyone who is too poor, too busy, too Black, too feminine, too queer, and too gender nonconforming, among others. The Autistics who lack access to fair diagnoses need solidarity and justice the most desperately out of all of us, and we can't just shut them out.*

When I first wrote my essay for *Cup of Jo*, I didn't understand the validity of allowing autistic people to self-diagnose. Had I understood, I might not have spiraled so quickly in the face of caregiver anger. While the second opinion from Sarah Hendrickx added a layer of iron and steel to the armor protecting me from internet opinions, it was ultimately nothing but time and research that made me feel comfortable in it.

I read essays and books, listened to podcasts, interviewed doctors, and, through it all, realized I would never be able to convince the parent brigade or the uninformed psychiatrists or the well-meaning acquaintances who squinted at me and said, "Yeah, but aren't we *all* a little bit autistic?"

What I really needed was to believe Dr. Marsh and absorb her wise words into my bones. "I trust you and your interpretation of yourself."

For so long I'd been waiting for someone to see me. Family. Doctors. Partners. Friends. But finally, perhaps for the very first time, I could clearly see myself.

—20—

Visible

IF YOU'VE EVER READ FANTASY OR OLD-TIMEY FAIRY TALES, AT SOME point you've probably encountered the idea of a "true name," a symbol of a person's deepest self that must be guarded closely, lest its power dissipate. Rumpelstiltskin, Voldemort, or Ged from *A Wizard of Earthsea*. Hell, even your mother using your full name to yell at you when she's angry: "Marian Lee Schembari Negroni, get in the kitchen this instant and clean your spit off the floor!"

This trope is a warning. Keep your identity secret, or it will be used against you.

At thirty-four, I discovered that no power grows while cowering in the dark. Learning and sharing the word *autism* would heal decades of wounds. Dozens of relationships. A lifetime of self-hatred. Six letters gave language to the terrain of my life. I could read the original transcript of myself, now a palimpsest of every person I'd ever tried to be.

The Centers for Disease Control and Prevention estimates that about one in thirty-six people is autistic. That said, we know autism goes undiagnosed in marginalized genders and people of color, so we can assume this number to be significantly higher. Women like me are being diagnosed every day. We are everywhere, hiding in plain sight, wearing the masks we were given as children.

My heart aches for them, and for her—the Marian who begged to be changed at nine and nineteen, who ran into classroom closets and office bathrooms. "Someday," I would tell her, "you will have a name for what you are. And you will never again have to keep it hidden."

IT'S BEEN THREE YEARS since my diagnosis. Last Christmas, the entire Schembari Negroni family was back in Old Greenwich, and the house was drooping under the weight of the partners and pets and children we'd amassed over the years: eleven people, two dogs, and two cats cooped up in the colorful house next to the woods.

"While you're here," Mom said, "I'd love to grab some alone time with you."

We were sitting across from June at the kitchen table of my childhood, where she was eating bright-blue Cookie Monster ice cream in the dead of winter.

I cocked my head. "Sure?"

"I've been thinking a lot about your diagnosis," she elaborated, "and whether I should have known. I've been kicking myself for not seeing it."

I opened my mouth to absolve her, but before I could say anything she added, "Not now." She side-eyed June, whose mouth was fully turquoise. "When we can really talk."

The previous fall I'd blurted out *Iwasdiagnosedwithautism* in the hygiene aisle of a health food store in Ohio, where we were gathered for Antonio's wedding.

Her eyes had shot up to mine from a paper box of compostable dental floss.

"What does that mean?" she asked.

I struggled to find the words. "Oh, you know, social anxiety, sensory issues like problems with itchy tags and stuff . . ." I trailed off, forgetting everything I knew about autism as we made our way to the checkout line, where the smell of rotisserie chicken and the sounds of five lanes of scanner beeps pulled at my attention.

"Oh, I have that!" Mom said. "The itchy clothes thing." She put the dental floss on the conveyor belt.

"There you go, maybe you're autistic." I laughed as if this were all a joke. If I could make it seem inconsequential, it would hurt less when she rejected it.

We walked back through the hot parking lot and got into her car.

"Can I tell your father about this?" she asked.

"Sure." I shrugged.

For over a year, she didn't mention it again, and I wasn't about to push it. I assumed she didn't believe me or didn't care or was brushing it off as one of my many moments of oversensitivity. Mom has no memory of this conversation and believes I simply emailed her a link to the *Cup of Jo* essay I wrote six months later. Either way, we didn't have a proper conversation about it until just after Christmas, two days before my flight back home to Portland, when I passed her in the foyer.

"Do you want to go for a walk this afternoon?" she asked.

"Yeah, great, I was thinking the same thing!" I squeaked, barely managing to hide my anxiety.

We drove to Bruce Park, where the grass was green and the trees were gray. The sky was such a vivid blue that you might have thought it was the height of summer, but the wind slapped at our faces and delivered a constant roaring in our ears like a divine hand rubbing across the top of a microphone. We stuffed our hands deep into our pockets and zipped our jackets to our chins.

Mom didn't waste any time.

"So anyway, I wanted to talk to you because I started reading about autism and watching some YouTube videos, because I am mystified as to how I missed it. And I've sort of beaten myself up a bit about that."

"I don't think you should beat yourself up," I said. "Nobody was catching girls back then." It was the truth. I didn't blame my parents for not seeing it.

Mom explained that she wanted to understand now. *What's the connection between autism and depression? How did you feel growing up in a house full of loud boys? What were your friendships like?*

We walked for an hour, following the paved, winding path around the Bruce Museum and passing a group of men blowing leaves into the howling wind. I told her how it felt to be called lazy growing up, and how broken I seemed in comparison to her and my merry band of brothers. I told her that when she expressed concern that I was noncommittal and unprofessional in my career, I'd been trying as hard as I could to make any one of my jobs stick.

When the weather became unbearable and I started chattering through my words, Mom led us back to the car, where I bundled into the passenger seat and stared out the window at the frozen pond. Mom's gloved hands sat folded in her lap. I could feel her gaze; the skin on my face itched in the places her eyes touched me. Then she spoke.

"I am so sorry," she whispered.

Her words were a magnet, pulling my eyes to hers.

"Sometimes I don't think you understand how much I love you," she said. "I do. I love you *a lot*. You know how you love June?"

I remembered the night my daughter was born, that moment I recognized her in the hospital and the pull to tuck her back inside me where I could protect her always. I thought of how I yelled at June even though I loved her so much it sometimes physically hurt to look at her.

I wondered what life might have been like for my mother had *she* known about my autism. Instead of struggling to parent a daughter who baffled her, she could have said to herself, *Ah, there's Marian stimming again with her hair. It's gross, but I know she needs something to do with her hands and mouth right now—maybe I can give her a lollipop. Or . . . I bet Marian is inside because the boys are too loud. I should just let her enjoy the quiet instead of forcing her to play basketball with them.*

"I love you like you love June," Mom said, interrupting my thoughts, her voice fierce. "I love you that much. *I love you that much.*"

She couldn't have been the mother she wanted to be because *she didn't know either.* I'm sure all she saw was this awkward, antisocial girl who sucked her hair and read books and refused to play with her brothers. I felt sad for her and this inability to know me until now.

"I love you too," I said quietly. She reached for me, awkward across the gear shift. I wrapped my arms around her thin shoulders and tucked my face into the crook of her neck. A bubbling leaped in my chest, almost like a sob or a laugh. Maybe it was hope. Maybe it was safety—a full-body release into someone else taking care of you.

Mom patted my back, then pulled away.

"So the bigger question is," she said, clearing her throat, "how can I be better now, as the mother of a woman who has autism, so that I understand you and give you what you need? Because I may not have done that when you were young and for that I apologize. But now that I know, I don't want to continue to make the mistakes that I made."

It was the perfect question. I didn't have a good answer yet, but what a gift to have been asked.

THE YEAR BEFORE I spoke with Mom in the car overlooking Bruce Park, I had still been thinking about autism in terms of living in a closet—bigger than the one in Mr. Bacon's fourth-grade classroom, with a soft couch and room for my family and the occasional visitor who wanted to pop in for some tandem knitting. The closet in my imagination was based on the dressing room at my brother Antonio's wedding.

The wedding was big and loud and lasted late into the night. At some point my heart had been replaced by a subwoofer and it banged against the wall of my chest. My aunt, in a floor-length satin gown, waved me over to our family table, and she was saying something, but all I saw were moving lips, as if I were listening underwater. I could sense the beginnings of a shutdown, so I walked toward the small dressing room off the main dance floor, which had a door that closed and a cushy leather couch pushed against the wall.

As the door shut behind me, I broke through the surface. The bass still thumped outside but it was softer in here. I kicked off my heels and lay on the couch with my head resting on the arm.

The sounds of a party bleeding through a door had always served as an unwelcome reminder that people were enjoying life without me, but that night I was comforted by its muffled presence, like the beat of a lover's heart through their shirt. *That's my family out there*, I thought warmly. *My husband and daughter. My new sister.*

The door cracked open, and Elliot appeared around the frame, tie loosened and suit jacket slung over one arm.

"Can I join you?" he asked.

"Yes please." I lifted my head so he could sit, before resting it back on his warm lap.

"You need anything?" he asked, petting my hair. My eyes drifted closed.

"I'm fine," I muttered. "I'm lying here waiting to feel like a sensitive moody broken loser for running away from my brother's wedding, for not being able to stay"—I waved at the door—"out there. But I don't."

"That's great," he said. We settled into silence, listening to the party together in this tiny room.

We stayed there the rest of the night, and occasionally someone popped up to the surface with us. My sister-in-law Jenae wandered in, her wedding dress a cloud around her, just to quietly mess around on her phone. Then Brittany, the wild, extroverted bridesmaid, came tumbling in to grab her flip-flops.

"Are you okay?" Brittany asked, finding me half asleep on the dressing room couch.

"Totally fine," I reassured her. "It's too stimulating out there, but how great to have this cozy place to hang out."

"Cool," she said, already halfway out the door.

Sometime around nine o'clock, the door opened one last time and the sound rushed in along with four-year-old June, covered head to toe in bright glow stick jewelry—a two-tone neon headband, three slung around her neck, and another dozen stacked on her wrists. She looked like a bioluminescent fish.

"Hi, Mommy!" she said. She was flushed and beaming. I hadn't seen her for hours.

"What are you doing out there?" I asked.

"Just dancing. Okay, bye!" And with that she was gone, back out into the wild sea.

AFTER MY DIAGNOSIS, the closet had become a comfort. I finally understood why I retreated there, and that was enough for a while. But it was still *a closet*, the place you stuff old puzzles and mismatched gloves and muddy rain boots that no longer fit. A closet is not the place to live a life.

Once Mom asked how she could help, I started wondering what it might look like to exist in the world as part of a community instead of peering out between the slats of a door.

I called my cousin Lorea, the one with the silky hair who never complained about having it brushed. Lorea recently found out she has ADHD. When I told her about my sensory overload, she knew *exactly* what I meant.

"It's like the teacher from Charlie Brown," she told me. "*Wah wah wah wah.*"

Lorea and I talked about patience and rage and clothing preferences, about our grandparents and other family members who'd probably been neurodivergent all along too. After thirty minutes or so, we moved back into pleasantries, which were stilted, with long awkward pauses. What had been a joyful, enriching call was turning into a chore. I was ready to be done talking and I wondered if she was too.

"I hate the end of phone calls," I admitted.

"ME TOO," she shouted.

"I'm done talking now, but how do we wrap it up?"

"Did you ever watch *7th Heaven* growing up?"

"No . . ."

"Oh right, you couldn't watch TV. So on that show, whenever a character was on the phone, they'd just hang up when they were done. They didn't say goodbye. I always wished I could do that."

"That sounds amazing, let's do it."

She hung up on me.

It was perfect.

Is this what it's like to truly connect with other people?

Over the next few months, I called Natalie, my roommate from Spain, who I hadn't spoken to in twenty years; and Chelsea, who teaches Pilates in Hawaii; and even Lewis, who lives in Australia now with his partner and daughter. He and I talked about our time together in New Zealand. I apologized for how I was with his parents, how consumed I'd been with my own fear and unhappiness that left no room for him, but he waved me off.

"I don't think I was great at supporting you during that time," he said. "I knew you were struggling, and I'm sorry."

He had nothing to be sorry about. Even without the autism,

sometimes relationships don't work out. But I felt it again: that opening, expansive sensation of being seen and cared for, exactly as I was. Maybe I wouldn't have to live in the closet forever.

WHENEVER MY FAMILY GETS together, we make the pilgrimage to Colony Grill, a post-Prohibition tavern in an old Irish neighborhood ten minutes from the Connecticut house where we all grew up.

Last Christmas, my brothers invited their high school friends to join us, the same guys I'd known since they wore Spider-Man footie pajamas and littered our house with Nerf bullets and candy wrappers. They now have beards and wives. I like them, but their voices are deafening. Colony is deafening.

Our table held seventeen people, and we sat waiting for our pizzas for over an hour. June was whining, trying to climb in Jenae's lap. Flogging Molly blasted through eleven trillion speakers. A hundred patrons talked and joked and laughed, rumbling across the open restaurant. For ten minutes I smiled and chatted with everyone, then I curled into myself, trying to block out the sensations. Thankfully, I now carry a pair of earplugs everywhere I go, so I popped them in and let my head plummet into my hands. I didn't care if I looked rude; everyone at this table knew who I was, and I accepted that this was how I needed to get through the night. But still, I wouldn't say it was *fun*. It's not how I'd choose to spend an evening. Even with the sound dampened, the restaurant still surged around me and I could feel the presence of every person in that room, touching the live wire of my skin. My eyes closed. I powered down.

Then I felt a touch on my hand. Mom was looking at me, her eyebrows drawn together. I tugged out an earplug to see what she wanted.

"Are you having a shutdown?" she mouthed over the noise.

I nodded.

"Can I take you home?"

Take me home?

I was five years old, and my mother was offering to bundle me in her arms, smelling that warm way only mothers smell, telling me in her own words that I wouldn't need to cry alone on the playground anymore; I wouldn't need to cower in the closet.

For a moment I considered waving her off and muscling through, but her expression made me pause.

Let her take care of you, I thought.

To be cared for means to be visible—trusting others to see you and not turn away. As Mom waited for me with that expression I'd never been able to read, the pieces of myself solidified, like I'd taken off Harry's invisibility cloak or Sauron's ring of power.

When people ask why I wanted a diagnosis—there's no cure, no reliable benefits, no single test—*this* is my answer. With a name comes community and care, self-compassion and forgiveness. I'm not invisible anymore.

There is so much I still don't know about autism—so much that doctors still don't know, that autistic people can't agree on—but at least today, for now, there is a name for the whole of my brain, the blood in my veins. I wish I'd known it years ago. I wish the people who loved me had known it years ago. Maybe then, I would have felt a little less alone. A little less broken.

Mom guided me from my seat and out of the restaurant, where the door swung closed behind us and the bustling noises evaporated. We were alone in the winter night, illuminated by a single streetlight pooling golden yellow at our feet. A car sloshed down the pavement. A lone man hummed by the intersection, but it was quiet enough to hear myself. We shuffled down the sidewalk toward the car, and I looped my arm through hers, feeling her warmth through her coat. I rested my head briefly on her shoulder. And then I let her drive me home.

Acknowledgments

FOUR WOMEN ARE RESPONSIBLE FOR BRINGING THIS BOOK TO LIFE. Without them, this story would have stayed tucked away in my heart. First, Delia Martinez Bowen, whose autistic coming-out sent me down a yearslong journey of self-discovery, forgiveness, and grace. Delia, without your bravery I would still be in the dark. Joanna Goddard gave me space to tell this story on *Cup of Jo* and was the perfect cheerleader and advocate as it took on a life of its own. Mollie Glick, my wise and relentless agent, emailed me after reading the aforementioned story and said, "I think you should write a book," which subsequently blew up my life and has allowed me to do the Thing I've Always Wanted. And finally, my brilliant editor, Lee Oglesby, who not only thought it was a story worth sharing but worked with me every step of the way, including parsing through endless spiraling emails where I changed my mind twenty-seven times. She laughed at my dumb jokes and helped make this book better than it could have *ever* been on my own. Thank you, Lee, from the absolute bottom of my heart.

Of course, there are a million other people without whom I could never have written this book, never mind turned it into a real live object you can hold in your hands and/or use as a coaster, doorstop, or cockroach-killing device. Jane Haxby, thank you for teaching me how to actually spell the word *toward*. Amanda Weiss, thank you for the beautiful cover. Morgan Mitchell, Jen Edwards, Mary Retta, and, of course, Bob Miller for your infectious enthusiasm during our first call. Cat Kenney, Christopher Smith, and Maris Tasaka are a marketing and publicity dream team.

For the editors and writers who mentored me over the years: Marie Forleo, Kate Moses, Lisa Jones, Allison K. Williams, Meredith May, and Laura Belgray. I could do this only because you did it first.

A huge, bowing-down thank-you to my whip-smart beta readers Kelsey Formost, Dana Miranda, Kate Suddes, Mrs. A., and my cousin Lorea Negroni Gillespie.

Thank you to the researchers, journalists, doctors, therapists, and fellow autistics who answered questions and read chunks of this book to make sure I got it right: Wendela Whitcomb Marsh, Sarah Hendrickx, Hari Srinivasan, Devon Price, Edith Sheffer, Eric Garcia, Steve Silberman, Ira Kraemer, Heather Filipowicz, Samantha Stein, Iris Warchall, Maia Szalavitz, Kristen Hovet, Beth Bleil, Keivan Stassun, Natalie Engelbrecht, Ludmila Praslova, Megan Neff, Marisa Chrysochoou, Dana Goodman, and Tasha Oswald. And for the autistic people I interviewed who wished to remain anonymous: Thank you. I see you.

For the women who took care of my mental health and physical body while I wrote this book, especially Jona Behrer, Sabrina Seraj, and A.W. These were the hardest years of my life, and without you, I would have fallen apart.

Being a parent with a full-time job while also trying to write a book means very limited time to eat toast for breakfast, never mind feel inspired or "tap into your creative flow." Betsy Cornwell of the Old Knitting Factory let me stay at her historic Irish cottage–slash–art retreat to bang out the first draft of this book. Betsy, I miss you. Take me back! Pamela Loring of the Salty Quill Writers' Retreat gifted me with a scholarship for a glorious week of writing on a private island in Maine. *Thank you* doesn't begin to cut it, so I promise to treasure that outdoor shower for the rest of my days. Thank you also to Hedgebrook for two uninterrupted weeks on Whidbey Island. My life's dream has always been to live alone in a cottage in the woods like some literary witch. Thank you thank you thank you.

For Kelsey Formost, once again, who was not just a beta reader but also my emotional support silly little person. Thank you for taking my many frantic phone calls, for brainstorming in the car, for your edits and your enthusiastic support. And Muffin, the first person to make me feel at home. I'm sorry I acted like such a freak. Thank you for still loving me.

For my siblings, Antonio, Sam, Joe, and Jenae. I love you weirdos. And my in-laws, Bob and Tomi Speed. Ditto. My parents, who were talented, formidable writers before I was even a glimmer on the horizon: Jim Schembari and Christine Negroni. Thank you for your editorial notes, your open-mindedness, your attempts to see and learn, for loud family holidays and Garden Catering gift cards and flights across the country. I love you very much. And for my beautiful grandmother, Marietta Schembari, who died at ninety-eight shortly before she could see this book on shelves: I will always love you a bushel and a peck.

It would also be irresponsible not to thank my front porch with the kiwi vine and the shimmering jade hummingbirds who visit the overgrown fuchsia. Thank you to the fireplace that kept me company on dark mornings when I was frantically trying to write in a single stolen hour before starting the daily hamster wheel of parenting and work. Thank you to milky black tea and Yoga Refuge and rockhounding and knitting and fresh sungold tomatoes from my garden.

Last but certainly not least, thank you to my sweet family. My husband, Elliot Speed, is my own personal life coach and punch-up writer. He endured endless nights listening to me ramble about memoir structure. He read countless drafts and did all the dishes, school pickups, and turkey sandwich assembly. Most important, he was the first person to truly see me. You're the best person on the planet, Pickle. I'm sorry for *actually* being the one who doesn't put the car keys back in the bowl.

And for our brilliant, affectionate, generous, silly, imaginative daughter, June. My peanut, my little chicken butt, my Juni Tunes. In the words of Mark Darcy, "I like you, very much, just as you are." May you always see yourself clearly. I love you more than video games, sour candy, and the color green.

Notes

2: Third Wheel

14 *wrote for the* Bridgeport Post   Jim Schembari, "Treasures of the Heart and Home," *Bridgeport Post*, October 15, 1991.

3: The Rabbit

27 *Amelia Baggs in her YouTube video*   Amelia Baggs, "In My Language," silentmiaow, posted January 14, 2007, YouTube video, 8:36, https://www.youtube.com/watch?v=JnylM1hI2jc.

4: The Princess and the Pea

33 *an essay for the* New York Times   James Schembari, "When Brotherhood Is a Father's Dream Come True," *New York Times*, December 14, 1995, https://www.nytimes.com/1995/12/14/garden/close-to-home-when-brotherhood-is-a-father-s-dream-come-true.html.

38 *calls this sensory* pain   Ira Kraemer, "Autistic Sensory Pain and the Medical Consequences," *Autistic Science Person*, March 29, 2021, https://autisticscienceperson.com/2021/03/29/autistic-sensory-pain-and-the-medical-consequences.

38 *annoying, difficult, and "too much"*   Ira Kraemer, "The Spoiled Brat Stereotype and Autistic Children," *Autistic Science Person*, July 17, 2020, https://autisticscienceperson.com/2020/07/17/the-spoiled-brat-stereotype-and-autistic-children.

39   *The Intense World Theory of autism*   Kamila Markram and Henry
      Markram, "The Intense World Theory—A Unifying Theory of the
      Neurobiology of Autism," *Frontiers in Human Neuroscience* 4
      (2010), https://doi.org/10.3389/fnhum.2010.00224.

39   *Science journalist Maia Szalavitz*   Maia Szalavitz, "The Boy Whose
      Brain Could Unlock Autism," *Matter* (blog), Medium, March 11,
      2015, https://medium.com/matter/the-boy-whose-brain-could-unlock
      -autism-70c3d64ff221.

39   *"a quieter world . . . without the whine"*   Katherine May, *The*
      Electricity of Every Living Thing: A Woman's Walk in the Wild
      to Find Her Way Home (Brooklyn, NY: Melville House Publishing,
      2021), 381.

40   *adjusting to a stimulus over time*   Rebecca P. Lawson et al., "A
      Striking Reduction of Simple Loudness Adaptation in Autism,"
      Scientific Reports 5, no. 16157 (2015), https://doi.org/10.1038
      /srep16157.

5: Eggshells

47   *"Have you ever when sending an email"*   Deborah Lipsky, *From*
      Anxiety to Meltdown: How Individuals on the Autism Spectrum
      Deal with Anxiety, Experience Meltdowns, Manifest Tantrums,
      and How You Can Intervene Effectively (London; Philadelphia:
      Jessica Kingsley Publishers, 2011), 115.

48   *"went into a full-blown, sobbing meltdown"*   Devon Price, *Un-*
      masking Autism: Discovering the New Faces of Neurodiversity
      (New York: Harmony Books, 2022), 93.

7: Copycat

77   *"I learned to ask after people's children"*   Katherine May, *The Elec-*
      tricity of Every Living Thing: A Woman's Walk in the Wild to Find
      Her Way Home (Brooklyn, NY: Melville House Publishing, 2021),
      97–98.

79   *our social network is "the most profound predictor"*   Elizabeth
      Dixon, "The Importance of Cultivating Community," *Psychology*
      Today, August 20, 2021, https://www.psychologytoday.com/us
      /blog/the-flourishing-family/202108/the-importance-cultivating
      -community.

8: Lazy Failure Slob

91   *"What every parent of a child on the spectrum knows"*   Steve Silberman, "Autistic People Are Not Failed Versions of 'Normal.' They're Different, Not Less," TED Ideas, April 4, 2016, https://ideas.ted.com/autistic-people-are-not-failed-versions-of-normal-theyre-different-not-less.

91   *only 41 percent of us graduate*   Lynn Newman et al., *The Post-High School Outcomes of Young Adults with Disabilities Up to 8 Years after High School: A Report from the National Longitudinal Transition Study-2 (NLTS2)*, US Department of Education (Menlo Park, CA: SRI International, 2011), https://ies.ed.gov/ncser/pubs/20113005/pdf/20113005.pdf.

92   *defining autistic burnout*   Dora M. Raymaker et al., "'Having All of Your Internal Resources Exhausted Beyond Measure and Being Left with No Clean-Up Crew': Defining Autistic Burnout," *Autism in Adulthood* 2, no. 2 (2020): 132–43, https://doi.org/10.1089/aut.2019.0079.

9: Foreign

102   *"No one sees you as an 'overly sensitive'"*   Devon Price, *Unmasking Autism: Discovering the New Faces of Neurodiversity* (New York: Harmony Books, 2022), 70.

10: Buzzkill

114   *Spoon Theory was created by Christine Miserandino*   Christine Miserandino, "The Spoon Theory," But You Don't Look Sick, April 26, 2013, https://butyoudontlooksick.com/articles/written-by-christine/the-spoon-theory.

11: Highly Sensitive Person

129   *"The description of someone who is Highly Sensitive"*   Kristen Hovet, "Opinion: Highly Sensitive Person (HSP) and Female Autism Are the Same in Some Cases," *The Shadow* (blog), Medium, April 24, 2019, https://medium.com/the-shadow/opinion-highly-sensitive-person-hsp-and-high-functioning-autism-are-the-same-in-some-cases-842821a4eb73.

13: A Little Bit Autistic

151 *"The hardest part throughout the trials"* Jenara Nerenberg, *Divergent Mind: Thriving in a World That Wasn't Designed for You* (New York: HarperOne, 2021), 163.

151 *Writer and photographer Kay Lomas* Kay Lomas, "Why Working Is Harder Than It Looks for Many Autistic People," *Mighty*, January 21, 2023, https://themighty.com/topic/autism-spectrum-disorder /working-with-aspergers-difficult.

152 *85 percent of college-educated autistic adults are unemployed* Nicole Lyn Pesce, "Most College Grads with Autism Can't Find Jobs. This Group Is Fixing That," MarketWatch, April 2, 2019, https://www.marketwatch.com/story/most-college -grads-with-autism-cant-find-jobs-this-group-is-fixing-that -2017-04-10-5881421.

152 *"The personality-focused job application process"* Ludmila N. Praslova, "Autism Doesn't Hold People Back at Work. Discrimination Does," *Harvard Business Review*, December 13, 2021, https://hbr.org/2021/12/autism-doesnt-hold-people-back-at-work -discrimination-does.

153 *"I would not change my son for the world"* "Frist Center for Autism and Innovation," Vanderbilt University, posted July 18, 2019, YouTube video, 3:32, https://www.youtube.com/watch?v=uab55GEe05g.

15: Normal

179 *the widespread myth that menstrual pain is normal* Maya Dusenbery, *Doing Harm: The Truth About How Bad Medicine and Lazy Science Leave Women Dismissed, Misdiagnosed, and Sick* (New York: HarperOne, 2018), 223.

183 *"If you lost weight, you wouldn't have this"* Maya Dusenbery, "Doctors Told Her She Was Just Fat. She Actually Had Cancer," *Cosmopolitan*, April 17, 2018, https://www.cosmopolitan.com/health -fitness/a19608429/medical-fatshaming.

183 *"My doctor felt that losing weight would help"* Rebecca Hiles, "I Had Cancer—and Medical Fat-Shaming Could Have Killed Me," Everyday Feminism, September 14, 2015, https://everydayfeminism .com/2015/09/medical-fat-shaming-danger.

184 *Women are diagnosed* years *later* David Westergaard et al., "Population-Wide Analysis of Differences in Disease Progression Pat-

terns in Men and Women," *Nature Communications* 10, no. 666 (2019): 1–14, https://doi.org/10.1038/s41467-019-08475-9.

184 *We die at higher rates from heart attacks*   Brad N. Greenwood, Seth Carnahan, and Laura Huang, "Patient–Physician Gender Concordance and Increased Mortality Among Female Heart Attack Patients," *Proceedings of the National Academy of Sciences* 115, no. 34 (2018): 8569–74, https://doi.org/10.1073/pnas.1800097115.

184 *coronary disease being the leading cause of death*   "Women and Heart Disease," Centers for Disease Control and Prevention, https://www.cdc.gov/heartdisease/women.htm.

184 *When men have chronic pain*   Anke Samulowitz et al., "'Brave Men' and 'Emotional Women': A Theory-Guided Literature Review on Gender Bias in Health Care and Gendered Norms Towards Patients with Chronic Pain," *Pain Research and Management* 2018 (2018): 1–14, https://doi.org/10.1155/2018/6358624.

184 *adverse reactions to medications*   Marius Rademaker, "Do Women Have More Adverse Drug Reactions?" *American Journal of Clinical Dermatology* 2 (2001): 349–51, https://doi.org/10.2165/00128071-200102060-00001.

184 *lab rats are overwhelmingly male*   Katie Hunt, "Lab Rats Are Overwhelmingly Male, and That's a Problem," CNN, May 14, 2021, https://www.cnn.com/2021/05/14/health/sex-biological-variable-research-science-drugs-scn/index.html.

184 *undiagnosed by the time they're eighteen*   Robert McCrossin, "Finding the True Number of Females with Autistic Spectrum Disorder by Estimating the Biases in Initial Recognition and Clinical Diagnosis," *Children* 9, no. 2 (2022): 272, https://doi.org/10.3390/children9020272.

16: The Keys

193 *boys were 4.7 times more likely*   Azeen Ghorayshi, "More Girls Are Being Diagnosed with Autism," *New York Times*, April 10, 2023, https://www.nytimes.com/2023/04/10/science/autism-rate-girls.html.

193 *In a 2020 analysis*   Matthew J. Maenner et al., "Prevalence and Characteristics of Autism Spectrum Disorder Among Children Aged 8 Years—Autism and Developmental Disabilities Monitoring Network, 11 Sites, United States, 2020," *Morbidity and Mortality Weekly*

Report: Surveillance Summaries 72, no. 2 (March 24, 2023): 1–14, https://doi.org/10.15585/mmwr.ss7202a1.

17: The Door

202   *most plans in the United States don't*   "Autism and Insurance Coverage State Laws," National Conference of State Legislatures, August 24, 2021, https://www.ncsl.org/health/autism-and-insurance-coverage-state-laws.

18: A New Rule

217   *Morgan Harper Nichols learned she was autistic*   Morgan Harper Nichols, "I'm Autistic," *Morgan Harper Nichols* (blog), February 21, 2021, https://morganharpernichols.com/blog/im-autistic.

218   *Maia Szalavitz wrote about autism and forgiveness*   Maia Szalavitz, "My Own Intense World," *Matter* (blog), Medium, January 2, 2014, https://medium.com/@readmatter/my-own-intense-world-d0ef22d74496.

19: Impostor

228   *the CAT-Q, a questionnaire developed in 2018*   Laura Hull et al., "Development and Validation of the Camouflaging Autistic Traits Questionnaire (CAT-Q)," *Journal of Autism and Developmental Disorders* 49, no. 3 (2019): 819–33, https://doi.org/10.1007/s10803-018-3792-6.

231   *best piece of writing on this topic*   C. L. Lynch, "'Autism Is a Spectrum' Doesn't Mean What You Think," NeuroClastic, May 4, 2019, https://neuroclastic.com/its-a-spectrum-doesnt-mean-what-you-think.

232   *Francesca Happé, professor of cognitive neuroscience*   Francesca Happé, "Why Fold Asperger Syndrome into Autism Spectrum Disorder in the DSM-5?" *Spectrum*, March 29, 2011, https://www.spectrumnews.org/opinion/viewpoint/why-fold-asperger-syndrome-into-autism-spectrum-disorder-in-the-dsm-5.

233   *"Hopefully, as research progresses, we will develop a more appropriate vocabulary"*   Edith Sheffer, "The Problem with Asperger's," *Observations* (blog), *Scientific American*, May 2, 2018, https://blogs.scientificamerican.com/observations/the-problem-with-aspergers.

235   *an average life expectancy of thirty-nine years*   Leann Smith DaWalt et al., "Mortality in Individuals with Autism Spectrum

Disorder: Predictors Over a 20-Year Period," *Autism* 23, no. 7 (2019): 1732–39, https://doi.org/10.1177/1362361319827412.

235   *rates nine times higher than neurotypicals*   Tatja Hirvikoski et al., "Premature Mortality in Autism Spectrum Disorder," *British Journal of Psychiatry* 208, no. 3 (2016): 232–38, https://doi.org/10.1192/bjp.bp.114.160192.

235   *six times more likely to consider suicide*   Lucas G. Casten et al., "The Combination of Autism and Exceptional Cognitive Ability Is Associated with Suicidal Ideation," *Neurobiology of Learning and Memory* 197 (January 2023): 107698, https://doi.org/10.1016/j.nlm.2022.107698.

236   *John Marble explains it best*   Eric Garcia, *We're Not Broken: Changing the Autism Conversation* (Boston: Houghton Mifflin Harcourt, 2021), 80.

236   *including my old home of New Zealand*   Lauren White, "'Burdens' and Borders: Disability Discrimination in New Zealand Immigration Law," Equal Justice Project, May 4, 2020, https://www.equaljusticeproject.co.nz/articles/burdens-and-borders-disability-discrimination-in-new-zealand-immigration-law2020.

236   *deprioritized for ventilators*   Liz Essley Whyte, "State Policies May Send People with Disabilities to the Back of the Line for Ventilators," Center for Public Integrity, April 8, 2020, https://publicintegrity.org/health/coronavirus-and-inequality/state-policies-may-send-people-with-disabilities-to-the-back-of-the-line-for-ventilators.

236   *Disabled parents face frequent discrimination*   Robyn Powell, "Can Parents Lose Custody Simply Because They Are Disabled?" *ABA GPSolo* 31, no. 2 (March/April 2014), https://papers.ssrn.com/sol3/papers.cfm?abstract_id=2645347.

237   *"These connections to the Autism self-advocacy"*   Devon Price, *Unmasking Autism: Discovering the New Faces of Neurodiversity* (New York: Harmony Books, 2022), 86.

20: Visible

239   *one in thirty-six people is autistic*   Matthew J. Maenner et al., "Prevalence and Characteristics of Autism Spectrum Disorder Among Children Aged 8 Years—Autism and Developmental Disabilities Monitoring Network, 11 Sites, United States, 2020," *Morbidity and Mortality Weekly Report: Surveillance Summaries* 72, no. 2 (March 24, 2023): 1–14, https://doi.org/10.15585/mmwr.ss7202a1.

About the Author

Marian Schembari's first byline was at age eleven in *Highlights for Children*. It was a poem about dragons. Since then, Marian's essays about travel, friendship, money, and love have appeared in the *New York Times*, *Cosmopolitan*, *Marie Claire*, and *Good Housekeeping*. At thirty-four years old, Marian was diagnosed with autism. She lives in Portland, Oregon, with her husband and daughter.